Fore: T5-DHI-696

Back Problems

Graham Yost

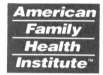

American Family Health Institute™

Medical Board

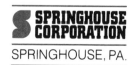

SPRINGHOUSE CORPORATION

SPRINGHOUSE, PA.

Program Director
Stanley Loeb

Clinical Director
Barbara McVan, RN

Art Director
John Hubbard

Editors
Jay Hyams
Susan Cass

Designer
Lorraine Carbo

Editorial Services Manager
David Moreau

Senior Production Manager
Deborah Meiris

Production Coordinator
Sally Johnson

The charter of the American Family Health Institute is to research and produce high-quality publications that enhance the health of individuals and their families. Essential to health are physical, emotional, and social well-being, not just the absence of illness or infirmity. The Institute's Medical Board has produced the *Health and Fitness* books to share up-to-date and authoritative information that can give readers greater personal control over their health maintenance.

Library of Congress Cataloging-in-Publication Data
Yost, Graham

  Back problems.

  (Health & fitness)
  Includes index.
  1. Backache   2. Back—Care and
hygiene.   I. Dudrick, Stanley J.   II.
American Family Health Institute. Medical
Board.   III. Title.   IV. Series: Health and
fitness series.   [DNLM: 1. Backache—
popular works. WE 720 Y65b]
RD768.Y66   1986   617'.56   86-5772
ISBN 0-87434-070-5

The procedures and explanations given in this publication are based on research and consultation with medical and nursing authorities. To the best of our knowlc·' these procedures and explanations reflect currently accepted medical practice; ertheless, they can't be considered absolute and universal recommendations. Fc individual application, treatment suggestions must be considered in light of the individual's health, subject to a doctor's specific recommendations. The authors and the publisher disclaim responsibility for any adverse effects resulting directly or indirectly from the suggested procedures, from any undetected errors, or from the reader's misunderstanding of the text.

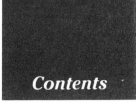

Contents

Back Problems

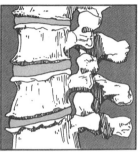

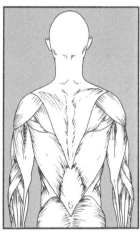

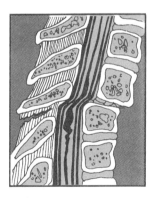

Your Back and How It Works

You can prevent most back problems by learning habits and taking actions that will strengthen your back and keep it healthy.

Your back is strong, resilient, and flexible. An intricate piece of construction, it's called upon to perform a variety of jobs. Your back allows you to stand; to walk; to bend forward, backward, and side to side; to twist; to lift heavy objects; and to curl up in bed. It supports the weight of your skull (heavier than you might think), your arms, your ribcage, and the rest of your upper body. And it performs another vital function—it protects your spinal cord, your brain's communication channel to the rest of your body.

As amazing as your back is, it can cause problems. Indeed, at any one time, some 80 million Americans suffer back problems.

The causes of back problems are many and varied. Some people blame evolutionary design for our back problems—they claim that the spinal column originally evolved to support people who didn't stand upright and walk on two legs. However, most recent studies indicate that our back problems result from our modern, sedentary style of living. This is good news—it means that you can prevent most back problems by learning habits and taking actions that will help your back stay healthy.

The first step in caring for your back is understanding its structure.

Sedentary
Sedentary means "sitting"—and most of us spend too much time sitting. Sitting puts even more stress on your back than standing. As we'll see (check pages 66 and 67), how you sit—even the chair you sit in—can make a difference.

The spine

Although sometimes referred to as the backbone, the spine isn't one bone at all—instead, it's composed of more than 30 separate, interlocking bones, called vertebrae. The vertebrae are separated by cushions known as disks. A channel through the interlocking bones holds the spinal cord and nerves.

The spine extends from the skull's base to the level of the hips. Viewed from the side, the spine is seen to have two prominent inward curves, one at neck level and one at the lower back. When we walk, sit, stand, or move in any way, the spine cooperates by bending, using these curves to cushion the motion. If the backbone were actually one long, straight bone, every jarring movement would be transmitted to the skull, which would be unworkable.

How the back muscles work

Two kinds of back muscles—those near to the skin surface and others in a deeper layer—let you move your back as well as your ribs, skull, shoulders, and upper arms.

The main superficial muscles are the trapezius and the latissimus dorsi. The trapezius, which are large, flat triangular muscles, connect the back of the neck, the shoulder blade, and the upper vertebrae. These muscles create the slope from the neck to the shoulder. Your trapezius muscles move your shoulders and upper arms. The latissimus dorsi are triangular muscles that extend from the lower vertebrae across the shoulder blades to the upper arms. They also help move these areas. A group of smaller muscles helps with these and other movements, such as lifting the rib cage.

The back's deep muscles keep your body erect. They extend from the sacrum and attach to vertebrae up the back to the base of the skull. Deep muscles are more numerous than superficial muscles, and their interactions are so complex that doctors often find it hard to diagnose or treat their disorders.

In addition to muscles, strong ligaments are an important part of the back. These flexible bands of fibrous tissue run the length of the spinal column from vertebra to vertebra, creating extra stability. They also help enclose and protect the spinal cord within the vertebrae.

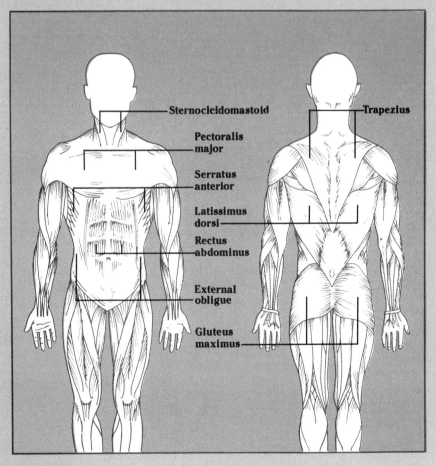

Sternocleidomastoid

Pectoralis major

Serratus anterior

Latissimus dorsi

Rectus abdominus

External obligue

Gluteus maximus

Trapezius

The spine is divided into five regions: cervical, thoracic, lumbar, sacral, and coccygeal.

The cervical section, composed of seven vertebrae, forms your neck and is extremely flexible, allowing your head to move freely.

Below the cervical section are the 12 thoracic vertebrae. This less flexible section serves as the anchor for your ribcage.

Below that are the five lumbar vertebrae, which are almost as flexible as your neck; they allow you to bend and sit.

Below that is your sacrum. When you were born, your sacrum was five separate bones, but during the first few months these bones fused into one, forming the back of your pelvis.

Your coccyx, at the bottom of your spine, is also known as your tailbone because it's all that remains of the tail we humans had in our distant past. Like the sacrum, the coccyx is rigid, being composed of fused bones.

Muscles may be the key
How your back feels is often a reflection of your muscles. Muscles support your back, and how much support you have depends on your muscles' strength. Sagging muscles won't support you adequately, especially when you give your back hard tasks like lifting.

Back muscles

Numerous muscles and ligaments are attached to the spine at various places along its length. The muscles move the spine when you bend, walk, or move in any way. The ligaments attach muscles to the bone. Of particular importance are the muscles attached to the lower back and abdomen. These support your lower spine during lifting movements. If these muscles are weak, they're unable to support the spine adequately—a major cause of back injury. Several factors can cause weakness in these muscles, including a sedentary life-style, poor posture, being overweight, improper sleeping positions, and incorrect lifting of heavy objects. Most back exercises are designed to strengthen these muscles.

Spinal cord

Your brain and spinal cord make up your central nervous system—the complex network of nerves that controls activities inside your body and your body's responses to the outside world. If you think of your brain as a computer, then your spinal cord is the conducting cable for the computer's input and output.

Understanding the spine

Typically, the adult spine has these vertebrae:
- *7 vertebrae in the neck area (cervical)*
- *12 vertebrae in the chest area (thoracic)*
- *5 vertebrae in the lower back (lumbar)*
- *5 fused vertebrae in the pelvis (the sacrum)*
- *4 fused vertebrae in the tailbone (the coccyx).*

Spinal disks connect the vertebrae, but the disks also keep the vertebrae apart. Each disk has a soft core surrounded by a fibre-like outer layer, shown in black.

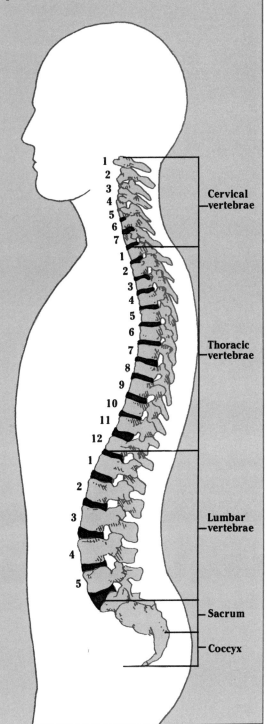

About 18 inches long and the thickness of your little finger, your spinal cord extends from the base of your brain down your body. Just as your skull protects your brain from injury, your spine protects your spinal cord. Your vertebrae form an interlocking protective canal for your spinal cord.

Nerves run from the spinal cord to all other parts of your body. These peripheral nerves are named for the four parts of the spine from which they branch: thus, you have cervical, thoracic, lumbar, and sacral

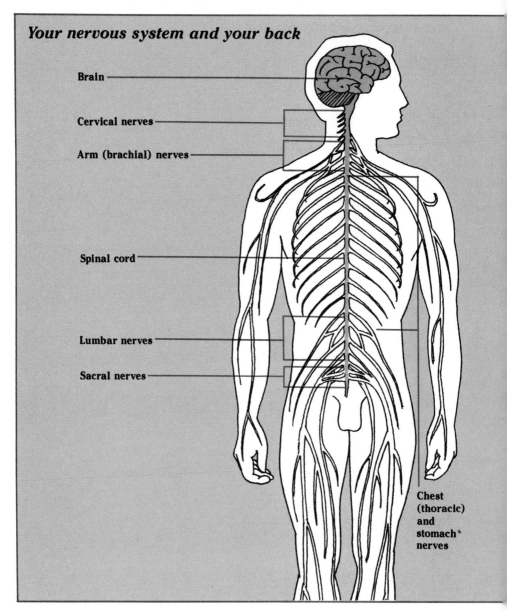

Your nervous system and your back

Brain

Cervical nerves

Arm (brachial) nerves

Spinal cord

Lumbar nerves

Sacral nerves

Chest (thoracic) and stomach nerves

peripheral nerves.

The spinal cord nerves and nerve roots (where the nerves connect to the spinal cord) are enclosed in a very tough, extremely sensitive material called dura mater. These nerves send a message of intense pain to the brain if they're ever impinged upon.

The spinal cord ends a few inches below your belt, at the beginning of the lumbar region. From there down, the spinal canal is occupied by a loose grouping of nerve roots called the cauda equina.

Your nervous system directs every body system and cell, controlling all movements, feelings, thoughts, and emotions. How? Its special nerve cells carry messages back and forth between the organs and tissues and the brain. For instance, if you accidentally put a hand on a hot stove, the nerve cells speed a message of heat and pain from your hand to your brain. Quickly, the brain sends a message to your hand to pull away from the stove. (These two messages travel a lot faster than your reading time for this sentence.)

Two parts of the nervous system make this communication possible: *the* central nervous system *(the brain and the spinal cord) shaded in gray and the* peripheral nervous system *(the nerves that supply the brain and spinal cord.)*

Certain peripheral nerves are called spinal nerves *because they stem from the spinal cord. The spinal nerves—you have 31 pairs of them—pass through very small notches in the vertebrae that protect the spinal cord. Any problem with the vertebrae, ligaments, or disks can irritate a spinal nerve, causing back pain and possibly pain in other areas that these nerves supply.*

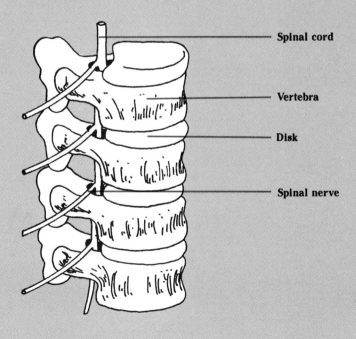

Spinal cord

Vertebra

Disk

Spinal nerve

Vertebrae and disks

Each vertebra is a thick, roundish piece of bone with several protrusions. These protrusions serve a variety of functions: some lock the vertebra with those above and below it; others serve as anchors for muscles or ligaments; and one helps form the spinal canal.

Between the vertebrae are disks—circular pads composed of a soft, jellylike interior enclosed in a tough, fibrous shell. Each disk is firmly attached to the vertebrae above and below it; the disk thus holds together the two vertebrae. Disks act as shock absorbers, keeping the vertebrae from grinding against one another when the spine moves.

All vertebrae are basically similar in design, with gradual changes as you progress down the spine. The two most strikingly different vertebrae are the two uppermost—the ones that support your skull. The top one of these is joined to the bottom one by a sort of ball-and-ring joint. This arrangement allows your head and neck to turn.

How the vertebrae stack up

This side view shows how the vertebrae and disks line up to form the spine. The disks connect neighboring vertebrae and protect them from each other. In the back of the vertebrae, the processes interlock. In the middle of the vertebrae, the holes form a tunnel for the spinal cord to run through. This tunnel protects the spinal cord, while allowing nerves to reach it through special notches.

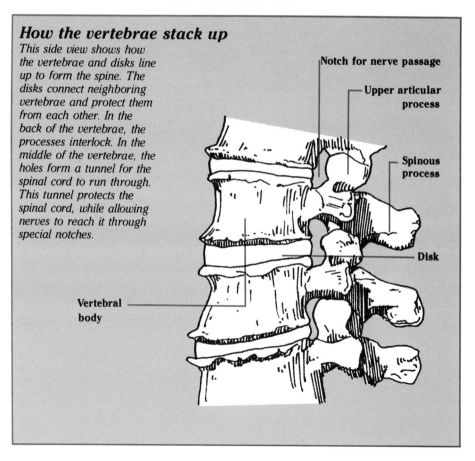

Notch for nerve passage

Upper articular process

Spinous process

Disk

Vertebral body

Parts of the vertebra

Basically, all vertebrae are similar in structure, but they vary in size, shape, and detail, based on their location in the spine. This bird's-eye view of a typical vertebra shows its three main parts:

Body. Located at the front of the vertebra, the body attaches to disks above and below it and supports the weight of the spine.

Vertebral arch. Together with the body of the vertebra, the arch forms a hole for the spinal cord to pass through. The sides of the arch, called pedicles, have notches that allow the nerves to connect with the spinal cord.

Processes. Seven natural growths called processes project from the back of the vertebra. Some attach to muscles. Others connect to the vertebrae above and below.

Vertebral shape depends on the vertebra's location in the spine and on the job it does. For instance, the first two vertebrae in the neck are shaped like a ring and a peg to support the head and let it nod and move from side to side.

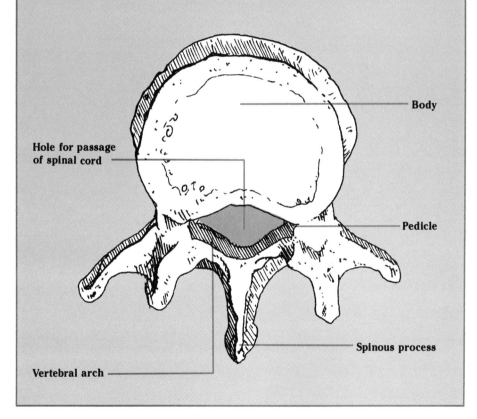

Body

Hole for passage of spinal cord

Pedicle

Spinous process

Vertebral arch

Vertebrae and disks are strong. Vertebrae don't easily break or crack; you can more easily dislocate your shoulder than dislocate vertebrae. Disks are even stronger and more resistant to injury than vertebrae. Even so, things can go wrong and create pain—the pain we call backache.

2 Back Pain: Natural Causes

E ven with their strength, disks are a frequent cause of back problems. The disks most often involved in back problems are those in the spine's cervical and lumbar regions. These spine sections are called on the most when you move, and the movement causes wear and tear. The thoracic region, supporting your ribcage, doesn't move much, so it doesn't usually cause trouble. Your sacrum and coccyx, also immobile, are rarely the cause for problems, except in certain types of falls.

A disk usually causes trouble in one of two ways. It can shrink, which reduces the space between the vertebrae, throws the facet joints out of alignment, and causes pain. Or it can herniate: the soft nucleus presses into, and sometimes bursts right through, the anulus.

Disk degeneration

Disk degeneration begins when you're a teenager, just after you stop growing. At that age, your disks are relatively soft and moist, but as you get older, they lose their moisture and shrink. If everything goes properly, this natural process of degeneration proceeds gradually and smoothly, and your spine adapts to the changes.

But degeneration doesn't always proceed smoothly and evenly, especially not in the disks exposed to the greatest wear and tear—those in the cervical and lumbar regions. There, the degeneration may speed up, causing a lot of pain. How? A shrunken disk may no longer completely separate the vertebrae it's located between. Then the vertebrae will rub against each other, causing small tears and bleeding.

Even if the disk doesn't shrink to the point where the two vertebrae rub, any change that the spine hasn't had time to adjust to will alter the alignment of the facet joints holding the two vertebrae together, and what once moved smoothly will now rub and grind. One little nick in a facet joint produces inflammation, which can make the muscles in your back go into spasm. The spasm stops you from moving and worsening the injury. Usually, the muscle spasm accounts for most of your pain.

Trouble spots
Specific disks in the cervical and lumbar regions are prone to problems. In your neck, the most common site for trouble is the disk between the fifth and sixth vertebrae; less frequently, the cause for trouble in your back is the disk between the sixth and seventh vertebrae. The disk between the fourth and fifth lumbar vertebrae is the most likely site for trouble; next is the disk between the last lumbar disk and the sacrum.

What happens in degenerative joint diseases

Usually you think of degeneration as a process of shrinking or wasting away. But as joints degenerate, ligaments and bones sometimes grow to try to compensate. You may have already seen this process at work in the finger joints of someone with osteoarthritis. Their joint problem may be so severe that they can barely bend a finger, but the joints themselves seem extra large and bony.

With degenerative joint disease in the back, here's what happens: injury, overuse, aging, and other factors cause wear and tear on the spine. This makes the disks shrink, and it flakes and cracks the cartilage that lines the vertebral joints. The body responds to the cartilage injury by trying to repair it. However, in degenerative joint disease, as in osteoarthritis, the repair process is abnormal. Instead, bone spurs—or osteophytes—develop at the edges of the cartilage, and the underlying bone becomes thick and distorted. Also, the ligaments grow and thicken, reducing flexibility and movement in the back.

The medical terms for this disease are spondylosis, degenerative joint disease, and spinal osteoarthritis. Although usually the result of a disk's gradual degeneration, spondylosis can also result from injury.

You can have spondylosis and not know it. You might not suspect that anything's wrong with your back. Then, as you reach across your desk for a paper clip, you feel back pain. That simple motion doesn't cause the back pain but is only the last bit of wear and tear that causes the microscopic wound, making your back muscles spasm.

Disk herniation

In a sense, all back trouble comes from degeneration. With herniation, the disks degenerate in a special way. Normal degeneration leads to disk shrinkage and loss of moisture; in herniation, something goes wrong with a disk's internal composition, allowing the soft inner core to bulge into or rupture through the tougher outer wall.

Herniation has three stages. In the first, the disk's soft core presses against the disk's outer walls. These walls, crisscrossed with nerves, send a pain message to the brain.

In the second stage, the inner core presses so forcefully against the outer wall that the wall bulges, pressing against a nerve root. The nerve root's covering sends a pain message to the brain.

In the third stage, the disk's outer wall gives way, and the inner core bursts through: a ruptured disk. In this case, the pain is compounded when the inner core presses against a nerve root.

Referred pain

Disk problems can cause you referred pain: although the source of the trouble is in one place, the pain seems to be coming from somewhere else. With irritated facet joints and first-stage herniation, in which the soft inner core presses into the outer wall but no nerve root is touched ("pinched"), you'll have referred pain. If it's a cervical disk problem, you may have pain in the shoulders and upper arms; a lumbar disk problem may cause you pain in the buttocks and thighs.

If a herniated disk presses against a nerve root, however, you'll feel referred pain all the way down whatever limb the nerve root serves. In the case of a lumbar disk, herniation can cause true sciatica, pain in the main sciatic nerve that runs the length of the leg.

What happens in osteoporosis

Normally, a group of hormones works to keep a constant level of calcium in your bloodstream. That way, calcium can travel to all the tissues that need it. If your diet doesn't supply enough calcium, these hormones remove some from your bones, where 90% of your body's calcium is stored.

If your diet is often low in calcium, you'll eventually lower your bones' calcium store, making them porous, brittle, and easy to break—a condition known as osteoporosis. As osteoporosis worsens, the spinal vertebrae begin to collapse, eventually leading to an abnormal curvature of the spine, sometimes called "dowager's hump," and possibly an aching pain in the back.

Who's at risk

Anyone can develop osteoporosis, but certain people—especially women—are at higher risk than others. (Osteoporosis affects about 10 million women in the United States, including more than a quarter of all women over age 60.) Here are the major factors that can put you at risk:

- white race
- fair skin
- slight build
- early or surgical menopause
- sedentary life-style
- family history of osteoporosis
- low-calcium diet
- therapy with glucocorticoids
- heavy cigarette smoking
- high intake of alcohol or caffeine.

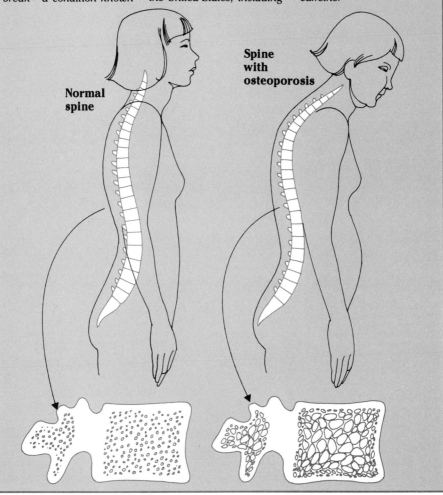

Normal spine

Spine with osteoporosis

Osteoporosis

Although usually very resistant to cracking or breaking, vertebrae can weaken. They can lose strength from osteoporosis, a degenerative bone disease that results from calcium loss, which makes bones porous, brittle, and susceptible to breaking. About one quarter of all elderly people suffer from osteoporosis, but women are three times more likely than men to develop the disease.

Most breaks in vertebrae weakened by osteoporosis are undetectable hairline cracks that require no treatment. Other breaks may be more severe and can cause great pain. Nothing more than rest is usually required for the vertebrae to heal, although in more serious cases a brace may be necessary.

The best way to avoid osteoporosis is to make sure you get around 1,500 milligrams (mg) of calcium daily. However, don't wait until you're older—the calcium depletion begins in your twenties. Exercise is also important because it helps bones absorb and keep calcium.

How to prevent osteoporosis

Here's how to help keep your bones strong, straight, and healthy:
• Get enough calcium in your diet. Make sure you have three servings of dairy products, such as milk, yogurt, and cheese, every day. To avoid increasing your daily calories, select low-fat dairy products. Or take the recommended amount of calcium supplements (around 1,000 to 1,500 mg of elemental calcium each day) after you've discussed supplements with your doctor. In some people, calcium supplements may lead to kidney stones.
• Avoid foods that are high in phosphorus. Phosphorus competes with calcium for absorption, so the more phosphorus-rich foods you eat—for example, meat, carbonated beverages, and processed foods—the less calcium your body can absorb.
• Keep active, and exercise regularly. Inactivity speeds up the loss of calcium and results in bone loss. On the positive side, exercise stimulates bone growth by increasing tension on bones and ligaments.
• If you are at high risk, see your doctor for early screening. If you have osteoporosis, he may recommend higher doses of calcium and treatment with sex hormones.

Kyphoscoliosis
In this disorder, the person has rounded shoulders, his chest protrudes, and his spine curves from left to right. The person will have no symptoms if his condition is mild. However, if it's severe, his heart and lung functions will be affected.

Scoliosis

Commonly known as "curvature of the spine," this potentially disabling condition begins at an early age. The curvature may be to the right, the left, forward, or backward.

The key to correcting this problem is early detection. Even children who appear completely normal should be checked. To check for improper alignment of the spine, the doctor will have the young patient assume several different postures. With mild scoliosis, a simple exercise regimen will correct the problem. More serious cases may require spinal braces or corrective surgery.

Lordosis

Excessive forward curvature of the lumbar spine, lordosis is a common back complaint. With too much curve, your spine's lumbar vertebrae receive too much weight. Poor posture and excess weight, both of which throw the curve even farther forward, can worsen the condition. Lordosis can cause backache and can accelerate degenerative back changes. Weight loss, posture correction, and exercise can correct lordosis.

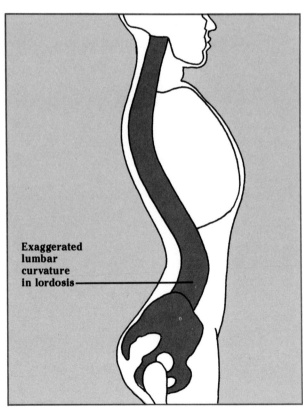

Exaggerated lumbar curvature in lordosis

Understanding and detecting scoliosis

A common childhood problem, scoliosis is curve of the spine. It can result from a birth defect, weakness or paralysis of the back muscles, abnormal spinal growth, different leg lengths, or even poor posture.

Normally, pairs of muscles and other structures keep the body in line, maintaining back posture and muscle tone. In scoliosis, the abnormal curvature puts a strain on the back's vertebrae, ligaments, and muscles, which leads to fatigue and backache. Without treatment, scoliosis can lead to restricted breathing (as poor posture squeezes the lungs), back pain, spinal arthritis, disk disease, and sciatica (from pressure on the sciatic nerve).

Fortunately, early detection and treatment can prevent these complications. To check for signs of scoliosis in your child, have him remove his shirt and stand up straight. Then look at his back and answer these questions:

• Is one shoulder higher than the other, or is one shoulder blade more prominent?

• When the child's arms hang loosely at his sides, does one arm swing away from the body more than the other?

• Is one hip higher or more prominent than the other?

• Does the child seem to tilt to one side?

Then ask your child to bend forward, with his arms hanging down and palms together at knee level. Can you see a hump on the back at the ribs or near the waist?

If you answer "yes" to any of these questions, notify your doctor. Your child needs careful evaluation for scoliosis. To correct mild scoliosis, the doctor may prescribe an exercise program. For more severe curvature, he may recommend a brace, a cast, or surgery.

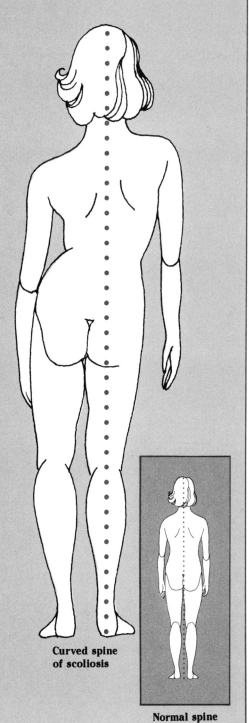

Curved spine of scoliosis

Normal spine

Kyphosis

Commonly called "widow's hump," kyphosis results from the degenerative process in which disks lose their moisture and shrink. As the spine gets shorter, an exaggerated curve can be produced, hunching the person's back. Although the condition looks painful, it isn't necessarily, because the spine adjusts as it slowly shrinks and curves.

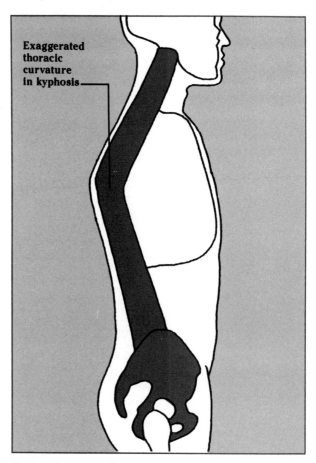

Exaggerated thoracic curvature in kyphosis

Spinal stenosis

Spinal stenosis is a congenital condition in which the spinal canal is narrower at one point than it should be. Spinal stenosis causes a problem when an overgrowth in the spinal canal at the already narrow point squeezes the spinal cord. The symptoms usually appear gradually and may include progressive pain, with or without a loss of sensation. A laminectomy—an operation in which a portion of the lamina (the bony protective enclosure of the spinal cord) is removed—can relieve the pressure on the spinal cord.

What's a "slipped" disk?

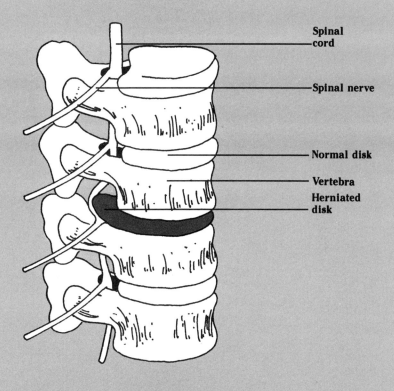

Spinal cord

Spinal nerve

Normal disk

Vertebra

Herniated disk

The term "slipped" disk is misleading. A disk can't "slip" because it's firmly attached to the vertebrae above and below it. When people talk about a "slipped" disk, they're actually referring to a herniated disk. Here's what happens:

Each disk has an inner core of soft puttylike material, called the nucleus pulposus, and a tough, fibrous outer shell, called the anulus. As the disk degenerates, the core tends to squeeze out—or herniate—through the weakest part of the shell, usually at the

back of the disk. When the core material bulges or leaks out into the spinal canal, it can press a spinal nerve against the small notch in the vertebrae through which the nerve passes. This can cause severe pain that extends down the leg.

Other back problems

The spine may malform in other ways. After birth, part of a vertebra may not fuse with the rest of that vertebra, which can cause discomfort later in life. Exercises to strengthen the muscles around the vertebra can help.

In another malformation, two vertebrae can slip slightly out of their respective positions, putting the spinal canal tunnels in the two vertebrae out of alignment. A small slip may cause arthritic pain; a great one may squeeze the spinal cord, requiring surgery to relieve the pressure.

Some of the rarer back ailments are just rarer instances of more common trouble. Cervical-disk rupture is an example. While almost all disk ruptures and nerve-pinching herniated bulges occur in the lumbar region, they can occasionally occur in the neck. Even rarer is thoracic-disk rupture. Because the thoracic region of the spine is relatively immobile, its disks almost never herniate and rupture.

Some other conditions and diseases—such as duodenal ulcer—can cause back pain, but such pain is usually referred pain: a symptom of a problem unrelated to the back.

Back Pain: Injury and Trauma

Most back injury comes from a pulled muscle or ligament. More serious injury comes from a bruise. The best bet for a sore or bruised back is patience.

Steve

Injury or trauma—a car crash, a fall down the stairs, a slip on the ice—can harm your back. Such injuries range from minor muscle strain and torn ligaments to serious traumas that injure the spinal cord, resulting in paralysis.

Muscle or ligament pulls

The most common back injury is a simple muscle or ligament pull. Perhaps you're in the park, playing touch football with some friends. You're out for a pass and you make a twisting, stretching dive for the ball. You feel no real pain right then, but later that night your back starts to knot up, and by morning you can scarcely get out of bed. If the pain passes in a few days, you've done nothing more than overstretch some muscles and ligaments. For relief, you'll probably need aspirin or another nonprescription anti-inflammatory drug and, perhaps, moist heat applied to the sore muscles.

Coccygodynia

The next most common injury is a bruise from an accident. You're walking down the street with an armful of groceries and you slip. You land hard, straight down on your tailbone—the pain is hard to bear.

This is coccygodynia, a bruised or cracked coccyx, and it's notoriously painful. In the past, doctors sometimes tried to remove the coccyx to stop the pain, but that often didn't work. The best bet for a spinal bruise is that most trying therapy—patience. (You can also bruise the spinous processes—the bumps running down your back). For coccygodynia, one of those doughnut-shaped pillows designed to take weight off the bruised area can be a great help for sitting until the bruise heals.

Whiplash

Perhaps the most common form of neck injury is whiplash. You're driving down a residential street, a child darts out from behind a parked car, and you slam on your brakes. The driver behind you isn't so alert and plows into your car. Your head snaps forward and back.

Whiplash causes strained muscles. Damage to ver-

What's a pinched nerve?

Pinched nerve

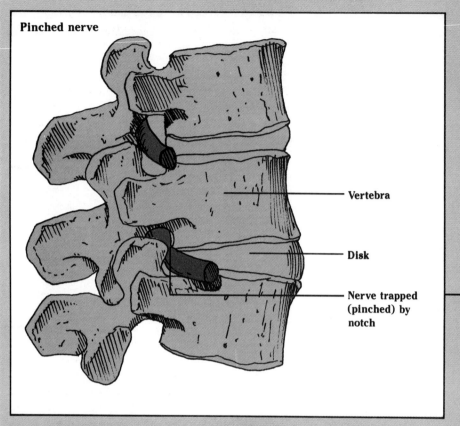

Vertebra

Disk

Nerve trapped
(pinched) by
notch

Normally, your spinal
nerves pass through a
small notch between your
vertebrae. This notch can
be a treacherous point on
the nerves' pathway to the
spinal cord. Why? Because
many conditions can close
off part of the notch, thus
trapping, or pinching, the
nerve.

The illustration shows
how swayback, a type of
poor posture, can pinch a
spinal nerve. Additionally,
tumors, broken vertebrae,
or a disk problem can
cause swelling in the area
or shift the vertebrae's
alignment and pinch the
nerve.

Normal nerve

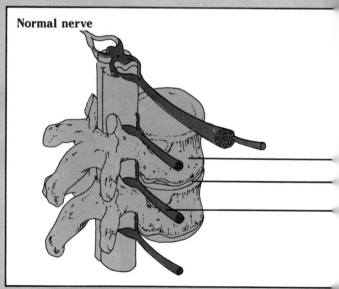

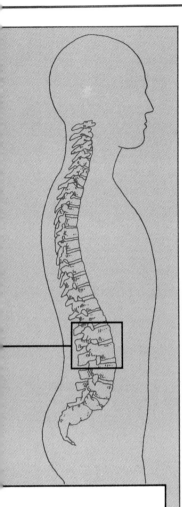

Vertebra

Disk

Nerve passing through notch

tebrae or disks is unlikely, and the pain should pass within a few days. A neck support or brace may help.

Emergency care for a back injury

In an earlier chapter we looked at what happens to your spine when it suffers an injury or trauma. For non-life-threatening but terribly painful injuries like coccygodynia and whiplash, emergency care involves lying down to rest the injured area and taking a non-prescription pain reliever.

However, if you've had an accident that raises any suspicion that you may have more severe back injury, answer these questions:

1. Do you have any back or neck pain or ache?
2. Do your legs or arms feel numb or tingly?
3. Are your legs or arms weak, paralyzed, or partially paralyzed?
4. Is your back or neck disfigured?
5. Is arm or leg movement painful?
6. Do you feel tenderness along the back of your neck or spine?
7. Have you lost bowel or bladder control?
8. Do you have difficulty breathing?

If you answer *yes* to any of these questions, ask for medical help immediately. Don't move from the accident scene unless you have to, for example, because you face further risk from a fire or explosion or because no one hears your call for help. Keeping still, if at all possible, is the cardinal rule of back emergency care. If something has been damaged, further movement could worsen the injury.

If you come upon someone else at an accident scene, ask the person the same questions you ought to ask yourself. If the victim's unconscious, you should assume his spine is injured. Send for medical help immediately and proceed according to these guidelines:

1. Again, move the victim only if he's in immediate danger.
2. If you have to move the victim, use a strong, rigid support—such as a plank, board, or door—to carry him on, so that his spinal position remains unchanged. You'll need at least two or three people to help you move the victim.

3. Have one person hold the victim's head, keeping it in an unchanged position. Don't let the head move forward or backward, roll from side to side, or twist.

4. Keep the person's head in the same position in relation to the rest of his body and roll him slowly onto one side. Slide the support under his body and then roll the victim back onto it.

5. Carry the victim carefully, keeping the support level and free of sudden movements and jarrings.

6. If you can't find a firm support on which to carry the victim, don't move him unless you have six people, three on each side, to carry the body and keep the spine aligned as you found it.

Many spinal injuries and traumas are treatable and temporary. Although much of the treatment is determined by the type and severity of the injury, proper care after the accident can help a great deal. The three cardinal rules are:

• Send for emergency medical help.

• Don't move the victim unless he's in immediate danger.

• If you must move him, keep his spine in the position you found it.

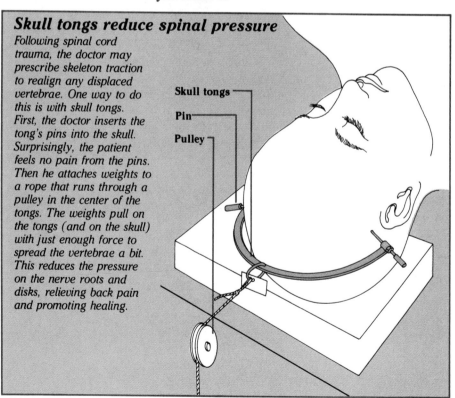

Skull tongs reduce spinal pressure

Following spinal cord trauma, the doctor may prescribe skeleton traction to realign any displaced vertebrae. One way to do this is with skull tongs. First, the doctor inserts the tong's pins into the skull. Surprisingly, the patient feels no pain from the pins. Then he attaches weights to a rope that runs through a pulley in the center of the tongs. The weights pull on the tongs (and on the skull) with just enough force to spread the vertebrae a bit. This reduces the pressure on the nerve roots and disks, relieving back pain and promoting healing.

Skull tongs

Pin

Pulley

Damaged spinal cord

The most serious form of neck and back injury is a damaged spinal cord. Among the many possible causes of spinal cord damage are a bullet, a car or motorcycle accident, and a fall while skiing. And every summer, doctors and nurses working in emergency rooms see victims who have dived into too shallow water and broken their backs.

Sometimes an accident victim escapes with a cracked vertebra, which heals after a few months in a cast or in skull tongs. Unfortunately, the spinal cord won't heal. As the body's main communications cable, once it's cut or damaged, it can't be fixed. A break in the neck can paralyze the body from the injured point down or cause immediate death. A break in the lumbar region can paralyze the legs. If the injury occurs in the cauda equina—the bundle of nerves that continues from where the spinal cord ends—the victim may recover if the nerve roots aren't injured severely.

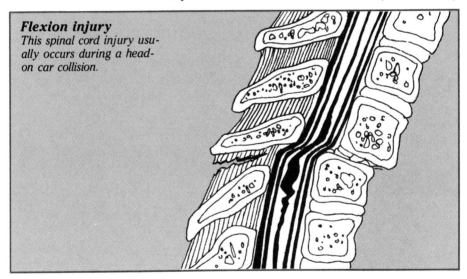

Flexion injury
This spinal cord injury usually occurs during a head-on car collision.

While people have survived airplane crashes and falls from burning buildings with every bone in their body broken but their back intact, others have been paralyzed by a simple car accident or a fall in the bathtub. So, although strong and resilient, your back needs your care and protection.

With injury and trauma that lead to pain, the cause of the pain is obvious. But with other back ailments—those caused by degeneration and herniation of disks—knowing the cause of the pain isn't always easy.

4 Identifying the Problem

Although back trouble's most striking symptom is pain, back problems can cause a wide range of symptoms from loss of full range of motion in a shoulder to loss of appetite.

Back trouble's most striking symptom is pain. The pain may develop slowly or strike suddenly; it may be a constant ache or occur only when you're in a certain position.

See your doctor if you experience back pain. He'll want to know certain specifics about your pain, especially its "what," "where," and "when":
- what brought it on (if you know)
- when it hurts
- where it hurts.

Your doctor will also want to know whether or not you're experiencing any other symptoms. In the case of an affected nerve, for example, you may experience a loss of feeling or a tingling in the arm or leg served by that nerve.

Back problems can cause a wide range of symptoms, from loss of full range of motion in a shoulder to loss of appetite. In spite of your pain, take exact note of how you feel and how your body is functioning. You may find that sneezing or coughing makes the pain worse, or that the pain occurs only when you bend in a certain direction. Such information can help your doctor diagnose your problem.

Your doctor's diagnosis

Today, a doctor can perform sophisticated tests to diagnose back problems. These tests are a recent development. Not too many generations ago, about all a doctor had for "technology" was what he could carry in a little black bag: a stethoscope, a tongue depressor, and a reflex hammer. To arrive at a diagnosis, a doctor would rely on medical knowledge and experience, what the patient reported, and information gleaned from simple tests he could perform with his hands.

Even with the great benefits technology has brought modern medicine, a doctor still relies, for starters, on what the patient says and on a few simple tests he can perform with his hands. Then, if he needs to know more, the doctor will look to the new machines to pinpoint troubles with an exactitude that was all but unimaginable as recently as 20 years ago. However, these tests are used most often for corroboration—

to confirm a doctor's diagnosis.

If you see your doctor because of back pain, he'll begin the examination by taking your history—how the pain developed, any other symptoms you may have, if you've ever had this problem before, and similar information. This can often be the most difficult part of the examination. Many people have difficulty accurately describing symptoms—even doctors, when they're sick, have trouble describing exactly what's wrong with them. You may find it difficult to describe your symptoms because your perception of your situation will be clouded by pain. Your doctor will try to guide you—somewhat like a detective questioning the witness to a crime—by asking you questions. The key facts he's after include the "what," "when," and "where" of the pain.

What? When? Where?

What brought on the back pain is very important. If the pain is the result of trauma—such as a fall or a car accident—its cause may be obvious to you. Pain that came on suddenly—after a seemingly trivial movement, for example—may indicate disk degeneration and facet joint irritation. Pain that developed slowly, over a day or two, may indicate a herniated disk, with the pain coming from an irritated nerve.

Asked when it hurts, you may truthfully answer, "All the time." What your doctor wants to know, however, is when your back hurts the most and when it hurts the least. For example, if you experience increased pain when you get up in the morning, the trouble may be the result of arthritic changes in your spine. If your back hurts when you bend over, you may have a bulging disk; an increase in pain when you arch your back might point to an irritated disk.

The "where" of the pain is often the hardest to pin down, especially if you're experiencing referred pain. For example, trouble in your lower back can produce referred pain in your buttocks or down the back of your legs.

Where does it hurt? Your first response might be that about all you know is where it *doesn't* hurt. That's a start. For example, if you have referred pain in your leg that doesn't go below your knee, your discomfort is probably not the result of a pinched nerve. The same applies to your arm—if your pain doesn't extend below your elbow, your discomfort probably isn't the result of a pinched nerve in your neck. True pinched

Another back strain
Being overweight adds strain to your lower back for the same reason being pregnant does. The extra weight in the abdomen tends to pull the body forward, and the back muscles must increase their tension to counteract the forward pull and keep you upright. The larger your abdomen, the greater the strain on your lower back.

If you have excess weight around your middle, try to reduce. Strengthening the muscles in your abdomen will help support the extra weight and take the strain off your back. See pages 50 to 58 for abdomen strengthening exercises.

nerve pain will extend all the way down one limb and only one limb, while irritated facet joints and herniated disks that aren't pinching a nerve can cause referred pain in either or both limbs—but never below the knee or elbow.

Symptoms other than pain

Your doctor will also be on the lookout for symptoms other than pain. For example, ruptured disks that pinch nerves can leave the muscles in the affected arm or leg either weak or feeling numb. Your doctor will check for such symptoms even if you haven't noticed them, because such symptoms aren't always easy to detect. And, of course, your doctor will be interested in any symptoms—such as fever or headache—that might indicate that something other than back trouble is the cause of the pain.

Your doctor will also be interested in your emotional state. Back pain is never "all in your head"—if your back hurts, it hurts. However, if you're under a great deal of stress, your emotional condition may intensify or prolong the pain. Your back muscles are the first part of your body to "tense up" when you're stressed, so if your back hurts, stress can worsen the problem. Not surprisingly, some of the worst stress comes from the anxiety back sufferers experience when they anticipate another attack of back pain.

Having taken your history, your doctor will probably have a pretty good idea of what's wrong. He will then perform a physical examination to confirm the diagnosis. The physical examination your doctor performs will be determined by what he believes is wrong.

If your doctor suspects you have cervical disk trouble, he may ask you to perform simple flexibility maneuvers, such as twisting your head from side to side, trying to touch your ears to your shoulders, and nodding back and forth. Your doctor will note any strained movements, and he'll ask you to report any pain you experience while performing the tests. He'll also test the strength of your neck muscles by pressing, alternately, against the front, back, and sides of your head and by having you hold your head steady against the pressure. Any significant difference between the strength of one set of muscles and another will give your doctor further information.

If your doctor suspects lumbar disk trouble, he'll probably ask you to sit on an examinination table

Physical examination
Your physical examination begins the moment you enter your doctor's office. He'll watch how you walk, stand, sit, and hold your head. Leg pain from pressure on a spinal nerve or a pinched nerve may make sitting uncomfortable for you, and you may unconsciously try to keep your weight off the affected side or you may choose to stand. Your doctor will watch to see if you limp while walking or if your toes are dragging—indications of a decreased ability to control certain muscles because of nerve root compression.

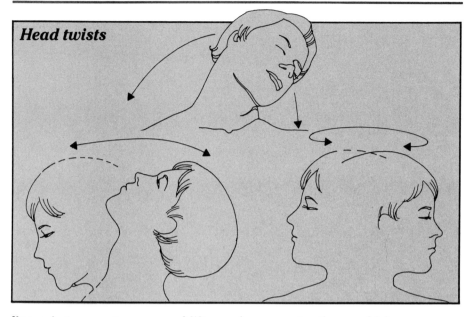

Head twists

If your doctor suspects you have cervical disk trouble, he may ask you to perform simple flexibility maneuvers, such as twisting your head from side to side, trying to touch your ears to your shoulders, and nodding back and forth.

and lift your legs, one at a time, as high as you can. The height to which you can lift your legs before experiencing pain will confirm whether or not you have a pinched nerve. To test the strength of your leg muscles, your doctor will hold your legs and feet in various positions and have you push against his pressure. If your legs are very strong, even weakened muscles will be able to move your doctor's hands. But if one leg or foot seems significantly weak, your doctor will again suspect a compressed nerve (on that side of the body).

To test for a pinched nerve, your doctor may ask you to walk first on your toes, then on your heels. If your calf muscles have been weakened, you'll be unable to stand on your heels.

The next test for suspected cervical and lumbar trouble is a reflex test. By tapping a tendon in your elbow, knee, or ankle, your doctor can provoke an involuntary muscle response—a reflex: your arm, leg, or foot will straighten in response to the tap. The reflex movement may be delayed—or it may not occur at all. Delayed or absent reflex movements may indicate that a pinched nerve is delaying or cutting off the message telling your arm or leg to move.

Your doctor may also stroke the sole of your foot. When the sole of a healthy person's foot is stroked firmly, the toes will curl down. But if the spinal cord or brain is damaged, the toes will spread apart, and the big toe will arch back.

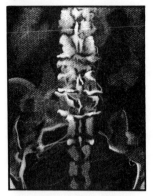

The doctor will probably order a spine X-ray if you have back pain, to see if any disk spaces are narrowed.

The last test, for suspected neck and low back trouble, is of feeling—the sensations in your limbs (hands and feet). Because of the many nerves serving your limbs, you may not notice if the sensation—the sense of touch—in your left thumb is a little weaker than the sensation in your right. But if the difference is great, from hand to hand and foot to foot, your doctor will have further indication that something is amiss with a nerve root.

Most of the tests your doctor performs are intended to rule out possibilities. What he expects to see is someone with back pain due to strained back muscles. Your doctor expects that you'll be able to stand on your heels, that your legs will be equally strong, that your reflexes will be prompt, and that you'll have full sensation in all your extremities. He'll expect back trouble that, despite your pain, won't require medical intervention—since only 1 patient in 10 with back trouble requires that kind of help.

In the vast majority of cases, your doctor will form a correct diagnosis of your back problem before you leave the office. However, he may need further tests to pinpoint the problem.

Tests with special equipment

One of the important tests available to your doctor—X-rays—actually dates from the early part of this century. X-rays, very short rays of radiation that pass through the body, are blocked only by bone. When these rays pass through a body onto photographic film, shadows of the bones appear on the film, allowing your doctor a partial look at the body's internal structure.

X-rays have only limited value in diagnosing back problems. They can pick up bony protrusions, malformed or broken (fractured) vertebrae, and spinal deformities such as scoliosis, but they can't see the real targets of interest: disks and nerve roots (although they can reveal disk degeneration when the space between two vertebrae has narrowed because of a shrinking disk).

However, a doctor can combine X-rays with the injection of a dye into the space around the spinal cord; then he'll see previously invisible areas. Of these injection procedures, the most used and most useful is the myelogram.

Myelography

To create a myelogram, a doctor injects a water-soluble dye into the fluid-containing part of the patient's spinal canal. Because the dye is heavier than water, the doctor can make it flow up or down the patient's spinal canal by tilting the table the patient is lying on. When the X-ray is taken, the dye stands out along with the bones. Any pressure, either on the spinal cord or on a nerve root, will cause the dye to gather. The dye will show the back problem's location.

Myelogram complications, while possible, are rare; and myelograms are 80% successful in pinpointing exactly which disk is pressing on a nerve root. Even so, most doctors recommend myelograms only when they anticipate the need to perform surgery.

Spinal X-ray showing injected dye

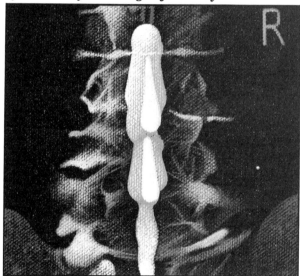

Discography

In discography, fluid is injected into the disk's core to determine how much fluid the disk will hold. A disk that holds a lot of fluid may be ruptured. However, degenerated disks have been known to take a lot of fluid; also, fluid can easily spill out of the needle hole and give a false reading.

Venography

Venography involves injection of a dye into the veins that surround the spine. The spine is X-rayed and the veins in an area where a disk has either bulged or ruptured should appear constricted. Unfortunately, this test is inexact.

Ultrasound

Ultrasound offers a more precise method of locating trouble spots. An ultrasound device transmits sound waves through body tissues, records the echoes as the sound waves encounter objects within the body, and transforms the recordings into a photographic image.

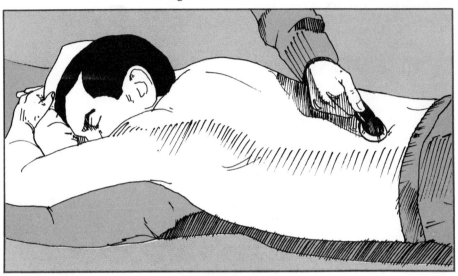

Electromyography

Electromyography tests the reaction of muscles to nerve impulses. A small electrical impulse passes fine needles inserted into an arm or leg. The results of the electrical signals are displayed as waveforms on a screen that an interpreter reads. Some waveforms indicate a muscle disorder; others, a nerve degeneration.

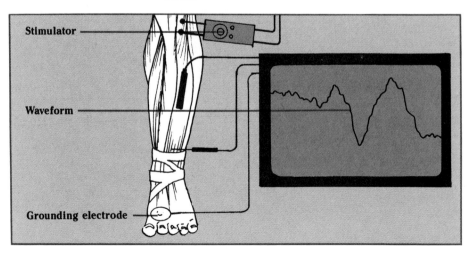

Stimulator

Waveform

Grounding electrode

Invasive vs
noninvasive tests
Invasive tests involve put-
ting something into your
body, like the dye for a
myelography or a needle
and fluid in a discogra-
phy. Noninvasive tests don't
cut or break the skin—no
physical invasion. Ultra-
sound is an example.

Invasive tests are always
riskier than noninvasive
ones, but sometimes they're
necessary. Your doctor will
start with noninvasive
"hands on" tests for your
back problems. If he plans
to do invasive tests, be sure
you understand what he'll
do and why.

Computed tomography (CT) scan

This test—the most revolutionary method for getting a look at what's going on inside a human body—joins computer technology to X-rays. Tomography attempts to improve on the simple two-dimensional pictures produced by X-rays. By taking a dozen or so X-rays close together—"slices," as it were—doctors can get a sense of depth by observing the minute changes from slice to slice. Computed tomography involves the use of a computer to study the slice: the computer picks up changes from picture to picture that are imperceptible to the human eye. What's more, the computer can join the information from the various pictures to produce three-dimensional views of a spine section. The computer image can be manipulated to show top, bottom, and side views of a spine section. The computer can also show things that were previously "invisible": disks and nerve roots.

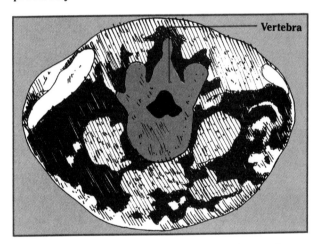

Vertebra

Although it is expensive, can cover only small sections of the spine at one time, and can't detect problems in cervical disks because of their small size, CT scans have been a boon to precise diagnosis. Combined with a myelogram, a CT scan can pinpoint what's wrong close to 100% of the time.

Your doctor may elect to perform other tests, including blood tests to check your bones and urine tests to make certain your pain isn't kidney-related.

The majority of these tests are used solely to confirm your doctor's diagnosis or to pinpoint the precise location of your problem. Your problem may not require the use of these expensive and time-consuming tests. Remember: the best diagnostic tools will always be your doctor's ears, eyes, and hands.

5

Treating Back Problems

You can treat back pain successfully— often with flexion (round your back) and extension (arch your back) exercises. With some problems, you'll need bed rest.

Great advances have been made in modern medicine during this century, from penicillin to microsurgery, but no cure has yet been found for a bad back. Even so, back pain can be treated successfully. A small fraction—about 1%—of patients require surgery; the rest need nothing more than bed rest.

Immediate care for back pain

Some back pain can come on without warning—as you reach for a pen or stoop to pick up some dropped change. A sudden racking pain strikes your back, as if someone has knotted and twisted your muscles. Other back pain can come on more slowly, starting with a dull ache that can build until it's ferocious after a few hours.

Back sufferers who've had repeated bouts with pain recognize certain signs of the pain's onset. If the pain builds gradually, they note a characteristic nagging ache that worsens. If their pain is more sudden, they develop a sense for the minor twinges that may precede the full assault. Back sufferers who know when pain is about to strike can use this awareness to do something about the pain. They can lessen its severity and in some cases ward it off altogether.

Their best immediate pain defense is the "flexion maneuver." "Flexion" occurs when you round your back, as when you sit in a chair and bend over to tie your shoes; "extension" occurs when you arch your back, bending it the other way. Both flexion and extension stretch the muscles in your back, but extension compresses your spine's disks and joints, while flexion decompresses them. Flexion can therefore help you at the first sign of back trouble.

If you sense pain's warning signs, immediately lie on your back on the floor close to a chair or a bed. Rest your calves up on the bed or chair, so that you can imagine a vertical straight line between your knees and hips. This flexion position stretches your muscles, takes the load of weight compression off your spinal disks and joints, and maintains good blood flow to your back. All these factors combine to lessen or ward off completely the painful muscle spasms

The flexion maneuver

Many back sufferers have found the flexion maneuver helpful in warding off backache. "Flexion" occurs when your back is rounded; "extension," when your back is arched. If you've had back problems, you've probably learned to recognize the warning signs of impending discomfort: a twinge, a building ache, stiffness. At the first sign of problems, lie down on the floor and rest your calves on a chair or bed. This position stretches your muscles, takes the load off your spine, and maintains good blood flow to your back. Maintain the flexion position for 10 to 15 minutes.

The flexion maneuver isn't restricted to preventing back problems. Many people find it a comfortable position to relax in at the day's end. When particularly bothered by their backs, some people sleep in this position, on the floor, with their legs up on the bed.

that cause the worst back pain. Maintain the flexion position for 10 to 15 minutes.

The flexion position does nothing to affect the pain's causes, whether it's a worn facet joint or a bulging disk. And, unfortunately, it won't work for every person for every back problem. If you're in pain's early stages and the flexion maneuver hasn't helped, then your immediate concern is to get home and lie in bed on your back.

On your way home, listen to your back. If you're unable to straighten up, so be it. If you have some mobility in your back, move into the position that feels the best—this will probably involve tilting your pelvis to remove any overarching. Once home, lie down, with your legs bent and your knees supported by pillows. You can use the flexion position—on your back on the floor with your legs up on a bed or chair—although you might not want to stay in that position forever, and getting out of it and into bed may be painful and awkward.

Call your doctor and let him know that you're having back pain. With his knowledge of your medical history, he'll advise you how to cope with the pain. Aspirin and other pain relievers will give a good deal of relief. A heated towel or heating pad placed against the painful area can relieve some of the muscle inflammation and spasms near the surface. If your pain is very intense, your doctor may prescribe a prescription pain reliever.

If the attack is severe, you could be on your back for days, even weeks, so you'll have some practical concerns. Arrange for someone to take care of your cooking and daily chores. Make sure that anything you need is within arm's reach. Get up only to go to the bathroom. Remember that at this point you won't prove you're "strong" by ignoring the pain. What takes strength is listening to your back and doing what it tells you to until it heals.

What next?
*You may wonder, while
you're in bed waiting for
your back to improve, what
you should do to avoid future back pain. The an-
swer? Exercise regularly.
Use the exercises on pages
46 to 63 to keep your back
strong and well.*

Bed rest

The best remedy for back pain is bed rest. Your doctor may advise you to stay off your feet for from two to six weeks, depending on the extent of the problem. This may involve having your meals in bed, using a bedpan, and receiving bed baths. It will certainly involve your patience, as well as that of the people around you.

Your bed should have a firm mattress (so-called orthopedic mattresses are probably best). However, if your mattress isn't firm, you can improve it by placing a board under it: a half-inch-thick piece of plywood will work well.

The doctor may also suggest using a heating pad to relax your tense muscles and aspirin or an aspirin substitute to relieve pain and reduce any swelling.

However, if your pain is severe, your doctor may prescribe a stronger pain reliever, a muscle relaxant, or an anti-inflammatory drug. Because such drugs can be addictive, you should use them for a limited time only; or, better yet, avoid them if possible.

Above all, you must remain in bed until the back pain passes. If you get up, you may ruin the treatment. If you try to ignore the pain and continue working, you'll only worsen the problem.

The only activity you should perform is traveling to your doctor for periodic assessment. If the pain doesn't go away after the prescribed period in bed, visit your doctor again—not all back pain will go away in a few days or weeks. If your pain continues, your doctor may refer you to a specialist for further examination and treatment.

Surgery

You may consider surgery the treatment of last resort—"If all else fails, I can always get an operation." Surgery, however, is only rarely the treatment of last resort for a bad back.

The success rate of back surgery ranges from 40% to 60%. This isn't because surgeons lack expertise; surgeons almost always accomplish what they set out to do. The problem has been that what a surgeon can successfully do may not accomplish the goal of healing a bad back.

Surgery is inappropriate for the majority of back problems because most are muscle problems, which don't require this radical treatment. Also, surgery is rarely appropriate in cases of back pain that result from irritated facet joints or even a herniated disk that is bulging and pressing against a nerve root. The case most likely to benefit from surgery is complete disk rupture, when a piece of the disk's core has burst through the disk's outer wall and presses on an adjacent nerve root. When a surgeon removes the piece of disk, the pain will probably go, too. Yet this surgery isn't performed frequently because complete ruptures of a disk, in which the core actually breaks through the outer wall, are quite rare.

Surgery can help only a small percentage of back sufferers. That's why more and more insurance carriers are requiring a second opinion before they approve the surgery. Even so, with one in four adults suffering from a bad back at some point in their lives, quite a number of cases each year are treated surgically.

An operation to remove disk fragments is performed under general anesthetic in a hospital operating room. The operation usually takes about an hour. With the aid of CT scans and myelograms, your surgeon already will have pinpointed the offending disk.

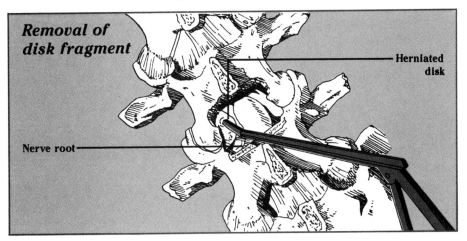

Removal of disk fragment

Herniated disk

Nerve root

With you anesthetized and lying on your stomach, your surgeon will make an incision from 2 to 4 inches long over the disk to be operated on. To reach the disk, he'll work as much as possible around muscles and ligaments. To gain access to the disk itself, he must remove part of the lamina—the part of the vertebrae protecting the spinal cord and forming the spinal canal. With a section of the lamina removed, the surgeon can see the affected nerve root and the disk fragment that presses on it.

Using magnification and special tools, the surgeon will remove the disk or pull out the disk fragment pressing against the nerve root. He'll then scrape out of the disk any remaining portions of the core to make certain no more of it bulges out. In time, the disk's empty center will fill with scar tissue. With the nerve root free and no longer compressed, the surgeon will sew up any muscles that he had to cut. He'll then sew up the skin internally—external stitches shouldn't be necessary.

Most patients experience pain when they awaken. However, this pain is from the surgery; any referred pain will be gone. You may have to spend a few days in the hospital, followed by a period of rest and care at home. With successful surgery, you should be able to resume your normal activities within 6 months.

Operations similar to that used to remove disk fragments can remove bony deposits that have built up (bone spurs) and are pinching a nerve root or the spinal cord. If the spinal canal is too narrow at one point and pinches the spinal cord, it can be widened by removing part of the lamina. Scoliosis is also correctable by surgery in which the spine is surgically realigned to remove the damaging curve.

Another operation for back pain that may be performed—although with decreasing frequency—is spinal fusion. Spinal fusion is performed to stabilize

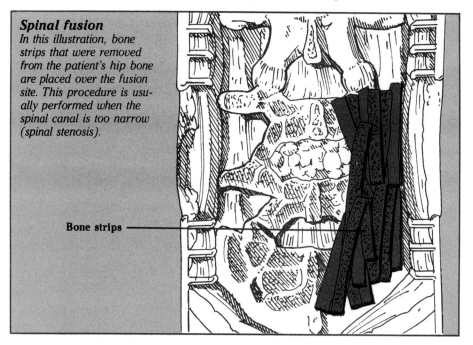

Spinal fusion
In this illustration, bone strips that were removed from the patient's hip bone are placed over the fusion site. This procedure is usually performed when the spinal canal is too narrow (spinal stenosis).

Bone strips

Back or front?

If the complete disk rupture occurred in the cervical region, most of the surgical procedure will be similar to the operation described here, but your surgeon may prefer to approach your spine through your neck instead of your back. Controversy exists here, over whether to operate through the front or back of the patient's neck. Surgeons who prefer to perform cervical disk surgery through the front of the neck insist they find fewer nerves, less bone, and no spinal cord to contend with. Surgeons who prefer the back approach say their technique affords a better view of the compressed nerve root and ruptured disk material.

a section of the spine. If, for example, the disk between two lumbar vertebrae has degenerated and is causing irritation in the facet joints, immobilizing those joints may stop the irritation and the pain. To fuse the two vertebrae, the surgeon takes tiny strips of bone, the size of paper matches, from the pelvis and attaches them to the vertebrae. A similar operation, known as vertebral separation, improves the separation between two vertebrae if that gap has narrowed because of a shrinking disk.

These two operations demonstrate the unfortunate distance between theory and therapy in dealing with back problems. Both spinal fusion and vertebral separation make sense in theory but don't always produce the desired result—the reduction of pain—and may actually worsen the patient's condition.

Because some surgical results are unpredictable, you should always get a second or even a third opinion if your doctor recommends surgery. Indeed, your doctor will probably urge you to talk to another doctor, and your insurance company may insist on it. Remember that even if surgery is appropriate, it may not be 100% successful. Conversely, if your doctor says surgery isn't the answer for you, and a second and third opinion agree, don't pursue the possibility of surgery. Unnecessary surgery is more than a waste of time and money—it's a dangerous example of overtreatment.

Overtreatment

Many back sufferers in search of relief run the risk of overtreatment. Pain, of course, demands attention. And you may become convinced that someone, somewhere, has discovered something new to cure your back problem.

The search for immediate and lasting relief can become a vicious circle, with the back sufferer going from one unsuccessful treatment to another. Some of these unsuccessful treatments may be harmless; others can be dangerous. Unnecessary surgery is the most dangerous type of overtreatment. A more common and more subtle form of overtreatment, also dangerous, is dependence on prescription painkillers.

Effective pain-relieving drugs can be invaluable during periods of unbearable pain. However, you can easily become dependent on such drugs, which is why most doctors are reluctant to prescribe them.

(text continued on page 42)

Drugs for back pain

Here is a list of the drugs commonly taken for back pain, along with a look at their minor side effects, serious side effects, and special concerns.

FOR MILD TO MODERATE PAIN

Minor side effects	Serious side effects	Special concerns
Acetaminophen (Datril, Tylenol)		
Upset stomach, diarrhea, dizziness	Liver damage, decreased blood cell count	Tell your doctor if you have liver disease.
Aspirin (Ascriptin, Bufferin, Cama, Ecotrin)		
Upset stomach, ringing in the ears	Hearing loss, stomach bleeding, slowed clotting, liver damage, allergic reaction	Tell your doctor if you have a stomach ulcer, a bleeding disorder, or liver disease. Take with milk or a glass of water. Stop taking the drug 1 week before surgery.
Codeine (usually Tylenol with Codeine or Empirin with Codeine)		
Constipation, upset stomach, drowsiness	Fainting, slow heart rate, liver damage, difficulty breathing	Drug dependence may result with prolonged use.
Ibuprofen (Nuprin, Advil, Motrin [by prescription])		
Upset stomach, ringing in ears, weight gain (from fluid retention)	Skin rash, hearing loss, stomach bleeding, liver damage, allergic reaction	Tell your doctor if you have a stomach ulcer or liver or kidney disease. Don't take *in addition to* aspirin unless your doctor tells you to.
Propoxyphene (Darvon, Dolene, Darvon-N)		
Constipation, nausea, dizziness	Confusion, difficulty breathing, liver damage	Drug dependence may result with prolonged use.

FOR MODERATE TO SEVERE PAIN

Minor side effects	Serious side effects	Special concerns
Dihydrocodeine bitartrate (Synalgos-DC)		
Oxycodone (Percodan, Tylox, Percocet-5)		
Drowsiness, constipation, dizziness, upset stomach	Shortness of breath, slow heart rate	Tell your doctor if you have liver, heart, or respiratory disease. These drugs can depress vital functions in the newborn. Tell your doctor if you are pregnant. Drug dependence may result with prolonged use.
Pentazocine (Talwin)		
Drowsiness, nausea, dizziness, constipation	Hallucinations, confusion, difficulty breathing	Before taking the first dose, tell your doctor if you have epilepsy or liver, kidney, or heart disease or if you've had a recent head injury.
Meperidine (Demerol)		
Constipation, dizziness, drowsiness, nausea, vomiting, appetite loss	Difficulty breathing, slow heart rate, fainting	Before taking the first dose, tell your doctor if you have liver or heart disease. Drug dependence may result with extended use.

Caution
- *Make sure your doctor knows if you are allergic to any medication. Be sure to inform him of any other medications you may be taking.*

- *Tell your doctor if you are or might be pregnant.*
- *If you are breast-feeding, make sure your doctor knows.*
- *Learn the potential side effects of the*

FOR MUSCLE SPASM

Minor side effects	Serious side effects	Special concerns
Carisoprodol (Soma)		
Drowsiness, dizziness, nausea, upset stomach	Allergic reactions, unusual (idosyncratic) reaction	Don't take this drug if you have a rare disease known as acute intermittent porphyria; call your doctor immediately if you experience extreme weakness or vision loss or if you become disoriented. Take with food if upset stomach occurs.
Chlorphenesin (Maolate)		
Drowsiness, dizziness, nausea, upset stomach	Stomach bleeding, decreased blood cell count, allergic reactions	Tell your doctor if you have liver disease or if you're allergic to aspirin. Take with food if upset stomach occurs.
Chlorzoxazone (Paraflex)		
Drowsiness, dizziness, upset stomach	Liver damage, allergic reactions	Tell your doctor if you have liver disease or if you notice a skin rash or itching. Take with food if upset stomach occurs. Medication may turn your urine orange or reddish purple.
Cyclobenzaprine (Flexeril)		
Drowsiness, dizziness, dry mouth	Low blood pressure, palpitations, allergic reactions	Tell your doctor if you have glaucoma, heart or blood vessel disease, an overactive thyroid, or problems with urination.
Metaxalone (Skelaxin)		
Drowsiness, dizziness, upset stomach	Liver damage, decreased blood cell count, allergic reactions	Tell your doctor if you have liver disease. Notify your doctor if a skin rash or yellowish discoloration of the skin appears. Medication may cause false urine test results in diabetics.
Methocarbamol (Robaxin)		
Drowsiness, dizziness, headache, upset stomach	Low blood pressure, allergic reactions	Tell your doctor if you notice a skin rash, fever, itching, or nasal congestion while taking drug. Medication may color your urine black, brown, or green.
Orphenadrine (Norflex)		
Drowsiness, dizziness, dry mouth, difficulty urinating	Palpitations, fainting, allergic reactions	Tell your doctor if you have heart disease or glaucoma. Notify your doctor if any of the minor side effects persist for longer than 1 to 2 days.
Diazepam (Valium)		
Dizziness, drowsiness, clumsiness	Extreme weakness, difficulty breathing, confusion	Tell your doctor if you experience any unusual reactions, such as extreme stimulation or excitement. Don't stop your therapy abruptly without first checking with your doctor.

medication you take, and notify your doctor immediately if you observe any of them.
• If you are taking a drug not on this list, ask your doctor or pharmacist to tell you about the possible side effects and special concerns.
• Take your medication as directed—take no more or less than the prescription calls for—and carefully follow instructions when you should take it and with what.

Get the cause of your back pain correctly diagnosed; get a second or third opinion.

The longer you use such drugs, the less effective they become at relieving your pain and the more you're likely to take.

Back braces are another form of treatment that may lead to dependence. These devices are used to give support to the back; some people, however, overuse braces and become dependent on them, which can weaken and further undermine the back's strength. Performing back-strengthening exercises may be the only treatment you need.

Avoid overtreatment. Get the cause of your back pain correctly diagnosed; get a second or third opinion. Remember that surgery is only rarely required. Avoid prescription painkillers—if you must use them, follow your doctor's instructions exactly.

Most back problems go away after adequate bed rest. However, the pain may return unless you take preventive measures. See your doctor when the pain has diminished. He or she will help you outline a plan to avoid future attacks. This will probably involve an exercise regimen along with some basic principles of back care—such as how best to stand, sit, walk, sleep, and lift heavy objects. Because no "pound of cure" is available for most back problems, an "ounce of prevention" is what you'll have to work with.

Recovery from surgery

All surgery stresses your body, so you must help your body recover by treating it with care and giving it time to heal. Most surgeons expect to put their back surgery patients on their feet within days and out of the hospital shortly thereafter. Your life should be back to normal after a few months, and after a half year, the scar should be about the only thing to remind you of the surgery.

For those first few weeks and months, however, you'll need to be careful. Much of this care is simple common sense. Obviously, you shouldn't overexert yourself. Don't lift or carry anything that weighs over 5 pounds and, if possible, arrange for someone else to take care of any chores that require moving things. For the time being, don't bend your back. If you have to pick something up or tie your shoes, bring yourself down to its level by bending your legs, not your back.

Follow the rules presented on page 65 about proper posture and day-to-day back care, only be even more vigilant. Remember that as far as your back is concerned, standing is more comfortable than sitting,

After surgery: Do's and Don'ts

—*Do* bend your knees when you need to pick something up off the floor.
—*Do* put your feet up on a footstool when sitting.
—*Do* keep your pelvis tilted back while sitting.
—*Do* sleep with legs bent and your knees supported with pillows.
—*Do* call the doctor if you notice redness or drainage from your back incision.
—*Do* ask your doctor for specific activity guidelines—for example:
  • *when you can shower or take a tub bath*
  • *when and what exercises to do*
  • *when you can resume sexual activity.*
—*Don't* lift or carry items that weigh over 5 pounds.
—*Don't* spend long periods sitting or standing.
—*Don't* ride in the car more than twice during your first week at home.
—*Don't* go up and down stairs more than twice your first week at home.

since standing puts less load on your lower spine, and lying down is best of all. While sitting, put your feet up on something to raise your knees above your hips. When either sitting or standing, pay extra attention to your posture, and keep your pelvis tilted back. When lying down, try to sleep with your legs bent, with your knees supported by pillows. Your doctor will tell you how many hours a day you should spend on your back. Follow his instructions closely.

For the first weeks of recovery, limit your activities as much as possible. Try not to ride in a car much for the first week, not only because sitting puts added stress on your back, but also because the car's vibration and motion may irritate your back. If you have stairs in your home, your doctor may ask you to limit the number of times you use them each day. Indeed, you should discuss with your doctor any and every activity you engage in, including when you can start taking showers and baths again and whether or not you should limit your sexual activity.

Because you've had back surgery, you'll have difficulty checking your incision site. Arrange for someone else to do it. If your helper notices any redness or drainage around the site, or if you feel pain or increased tenderness there, tell your doctor at once.

The other thing to remember, however, is that while surgery was traumatic for your back, which requires additional care for a time, your back is nevertheless quite strong and resilient. Follow your doctor's instructions closely and as soon as he says you can resume more of your regular activities, do so. Exercise is vital as you regain your back strength. If you want to achieve the full recovery that surgeons envision for their patients—where, after 6 months, the only thing to remind them that they ever had surgery is a scar—you must first be gentle as your back heals and then exercise and strengthen it to make it healthy again.

6

Exercises for Your Back

Experts disagree over some activities for back sufferers. Some feel the sky's the limit and that you should do whatever you enjoy, while others suggest that some sports can be worse than others.

Proper exercises are fundamental to the prevention of back problems. By performing these exercises, you strengthen the muscles that support your back and keep the joints in your back moving smoothly.

However, to give your back the best defense against trouble, you'll have to do more than just exercise this one body area. You'll need an overall fitness plan to keep your entire body healthy. (If you already have back problems, your doctor can tell you which exercises to do, which to avoid.)

Good sports, bad sports

Experts disagree over some activities for back sufferers. Some feel the sky's the limit and that you should do whatever you enjoy, while others suggest that some sports can be worse than others.

You can make your back sore rather easily, just as you can most parts of the body—for example, after carrying 2 heavy bags of groceries home 10 blocks, your arms will hurt (your back will, too). However, barring an accident, this tiredness doesn't injure your back.

Although some types of exercise are more likely than others to make your back sore, such exercises aren't likely to injure you—unless they're contact sports, which increase the incidence of accident and mishap. To decide which sport to pursue, use good sense. If the sport you love causes a little bit of backache but isn't dangerous to your back, perhaps you'll be willing to live with the slight pain for the sake of your enjoyment. If the pain isn't worth the sport, you'll want to choose some other activity that doesn't hurt.

Some noncontact sports are riskier for your back than others. Three types of activity put an added strain on your back: lifting weights, twisting, and arching.

Weight lifting puts an extra load on your lumbar disks and vertebrae. If you lift, be careful. Brace or support your back, bend your knees, and don't shift weight from your arms or legs to your back.

Any sport that jars you puts extra pressure on your lower spine. This includes all contact sports, horse-

Caution
Consult your doctor before starting any exercise program. Some of these exercises may not be appropriate for all types of back trouble. If you have the opportunity, also discuss these exercises with a physical therapist who can show you exactly how they should be performed.

The pelvic tilt

Master the pelvic tilt and do it wherever you are—waiting for a bus, walking down the street, sitting at your desk. You can do this exercise whenever and wherever you find yourself, and you should do it as often as possible. Doing so may seem awkward at first, but the more you do it, the more you'll get used to it. See pages 46 and 47.

back riding, dirt bike racing, and jogging (some authorities disagree about jogging and argue that jogging and running have never been proved harmful to the back).

Any sports that require the use of heavy equipment—such as toting a bowling ball or carrying a canoe—can also hurt your back.

Twisting motions are common in racquet sports like tennis, as well as in golf, baseball, and basketball. Sports that make you arch your back a lot include tennis and volleyball (in the serves), as well as hockey, rowing, canoeing, gymnastics, and skiing.

The pros and cons of sports must be balanced. Swimming is one of the best exercises for your cardiovascular health and is great for your back because the water supports you, keeping pressure off your back. Yet the backstroke will make you arch your back. Bicycle riding is also regarded as a great sport for the back. Yet the hunched-over position you may assume on a racing bike flattens out your lower back and can strain it, especially if you keep your head raised to see the road.

Avoid dangerous sports, particularly contact sports, and select a sport you really enjoy. If some aspect of the sport hurts your back, see if you can't deal with it. (For example, in tennis you might learn to modify your serve, and if you run, you might run only on grass or dirt.) Make back exercises part of your warm-up and cool-down. Performed conscientiously as part of your overall fitness routine, these exercises are your best bet for managing recurrent back trouble.

Exercises for your back

Follow these three rules when you perform back exercises:

1. If you experience any pain while performing an exercise, stop. The old "macho" maxim of sport—"No pain, no gain"—is crazy. If any of these exercises causes you discomfort, stop and tell your doctor.

2. For these exercises to do you any good, you must stick with them day in and day out. While they may be tedious, they're your best defense against future back problems. Look on these exercises as you do on brushing your teeth—part of your personal hygiene routine. (This exercise routine will take about 10 minutes a day.)

3. Always perform back exercises slowly and smoothly. Don't try to save time by rushing. Never try to overextend a muscle.

Most exercises designed for the back are variations or combinations of a few simple exercises to strengthen your stomach muscles, strengthen and stretch your back muscles, stretch and limber the ligaments that attach muscles to bones, keep your joints moving smoothly, and flatten out any excess curvature in your lower back. Exercises for the neck strengthen your neck and shoulder muscles, keep your muscles and ligaments limber, and keep your joints moving smoothly.

The pelvic tilt

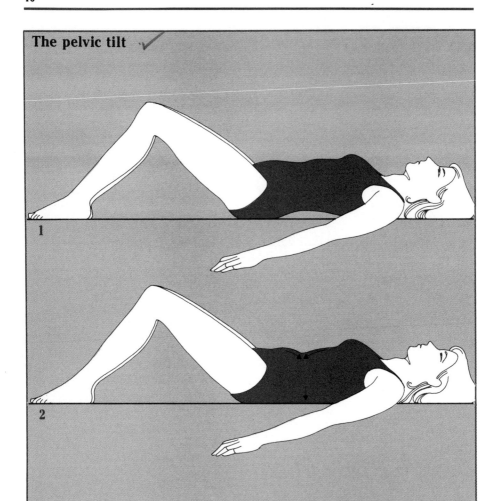

1

2

The basic starting point for most back exercises is the pelvic tilt. This exercise reduces the excess forward curvature of your spine's lumbar region.

1. Lie on your back on a hard, padded surface (a carpeted floor is fine); keep your knees bent and feet flat on the floor. You'll notice a space between your lower back and the floor.

2. Flatten your back against the floor; imagine you're pushing your belly button right down to the ground by tightening your stomach muscles and squeezing your buttocks together. These muscles will tilt your pelvis back, pressing your lower back to the floor and flattening out your arch. Hold this position for a slow count of six; relax, then repeat at least four times.

The standing pelvic tilt

1

2

After practicing this pelvic tilt variation, you'll be able to tilt your pelvis and flatten out your back wherever you are. A tilted pelvis is an important part of proper posture and this exercise is definitely worth doing.

1. Stand with your shoulder blades against a wall and your feet 6 inches out from the wall.

2. As if you were lying on the floor, tilt your pelvis by tightening your stomach and squeezing your buttocks. Tilt it back far enough so that the small of your back presses flat against the wall. Hold this position for a slow count of six; relax, then repeat 6 times.

The cat stretch ✓

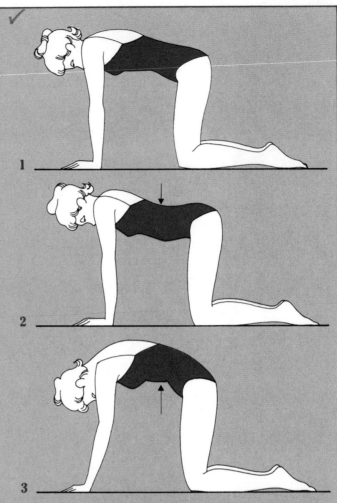

Stretching is an important part of keeping your back fit. Limber and stretched muscles are stronger muscles and will give you greater flexibility. This simple stretch is a good warm-up before your other exercises.

1. Start on all fours, with your hands and knees positioned at shoulder width.

2. Arch your back down, pressing your stomach toward the floor and sending your tailbone and head toward the ceiling. Do this slowly and hold for a count of six, then relax. If the movement hurts at all, don't push.

3. Now, arch your back up, rounding out your lower back and stretching your muscles in the other direction. Hold this for a count of six, then relax. Repeat this combination of the two stretches six times.

Rotation ✓

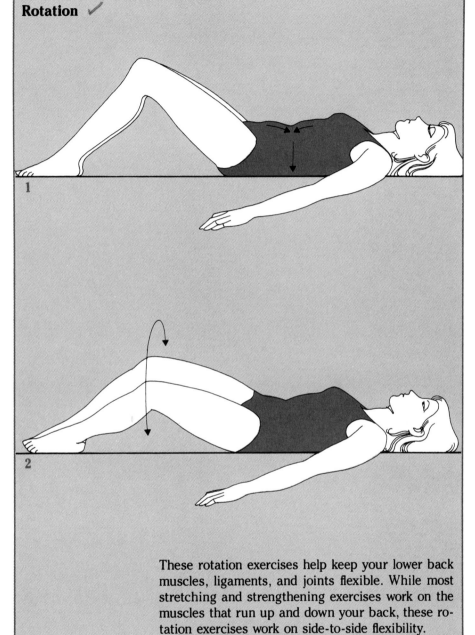

These rotation exercises help keep your lower back muscles, ligaments, and joints flexible. While most stretching and strengthening exercises work on the muscles that run up and down your back, these rotation exercises work on side-to-side flexibility.

1. Start on your back, with your legs bent and knees raised. Keep your feet flat on the floor. Use the pelvic tilt to keep your lower back flat on the floor.

2. Rock your knees from side to side as if you were trying to touch them to the floor on either side of you. Keep your shoulders and upper back flat on the floor.

Advanced rotation

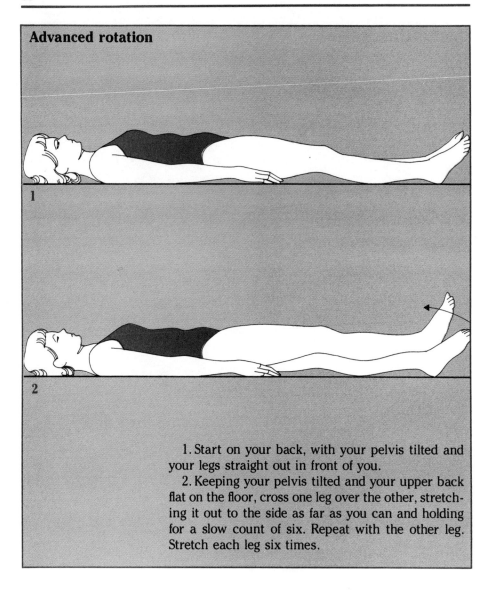

1. Start on your back, with your pelvis tilted and your legs straight out in front of you.

2. Keeping your pelvis tilted and your upper back flat on the floor, cross one leg over the other, stretching it out to the side as far as you can and holding for a slow count of six. Repeat with the other leg. Stretch each leg six times.

Abdominal exercises

The next eight exercises strengthen your abdominal muscles, which give your back the greatest support and strength. The exercises are in order of increasing strenuousness. Remember to maintain the pelvic tilt at all times through these exercises. And, for those exercises that resemble sit-ups, forget what you might have been taught in school—*do not* hook your feet under anything to give you better leverage. Exercises performed that way will strengthen your hip flexor muscles, not your abdominals, and over-developed hip flexors may cause back trouble.

The curl ✓

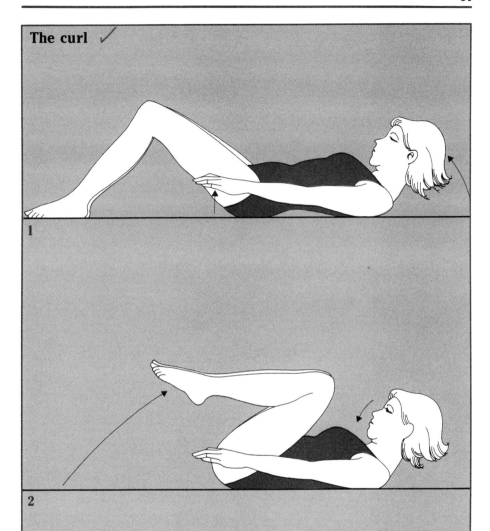

As well as strengthening your abdominal muscles, this maneuver also stretches your lower back muscles.

1. Start on your back, using the pelvic tilt, with your legs bent, knees raised, and feet flat on the floor. Put your slightly raised arms out alongside of you. Tuck your chin to your chest.

2. Slowly curl up, bringing your knees toward your chest and your forehead toward your knees. Go as far as feels comfortable, then uncurl and repeat six times.

Head and shoulder raises

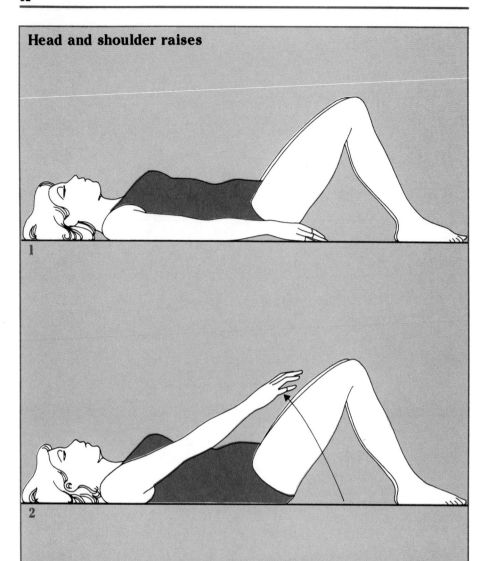

1. Start on your back, in the pelvic tilt, with your legs bent, your knees raised, and your feet on the floor.

2. Put your arms straight out in front of you and reach up with both hands to try to touch your left knee, raising your head and both shoulders off the ground in the process. Touch your knee if you can, then slowly lower your head and shoulders. Then try to touch your right knee in the same manner. Repeat six times for each side.

Leg raises

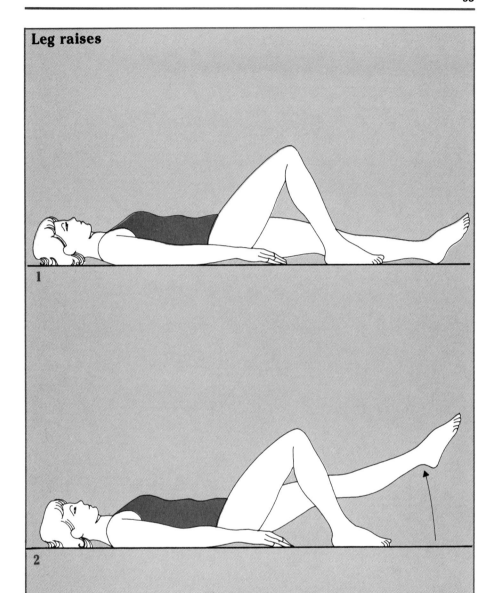

This stretches the muscles at the back of your hip and strengthens your abdominal muscles.

1. Start on your back in the pelvic tilt, with one leg bent and the other straight.

2. Keeping your straight leg straight, raise it to the level of your bent knee, hold for a count of six, then relax. Repeat this six times, alternating legs.

Toe touching

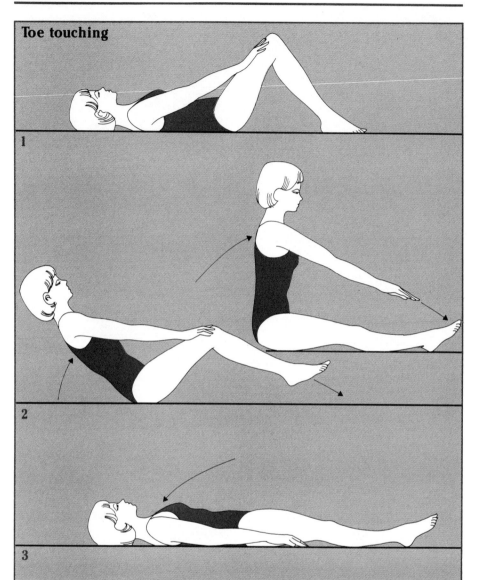

Remember to use the pelvic tilt throughout this exercise.

1. Start on your back with your legs bent, your knees raised, and your feet on the floor. Put your arms straight out and rest your hands on your thighs.

2. Slowly curl up, stretching with your arms, reaching for your toes. As you curl, straighten your legs and lower your knees so that, by the end, your legs are straight out in front of you as you stretch for your toes.

3. Slowly reverse the motion, uncurling, until you're flat on your back again. Repeat this exercise six times.

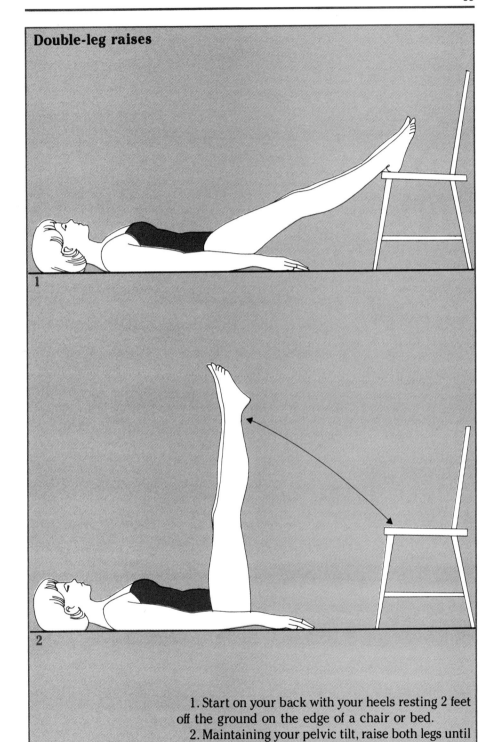

Double-leg raises

1

2

1. Start on your back with your heels resting 2 feet off the ground on the edge of a chair or bed.

2. Maintaining your pelvic tilt, raise both legs until they form a right angle at your hips. Then slowly lower your legs. Repeat this six times.

Sit-ups

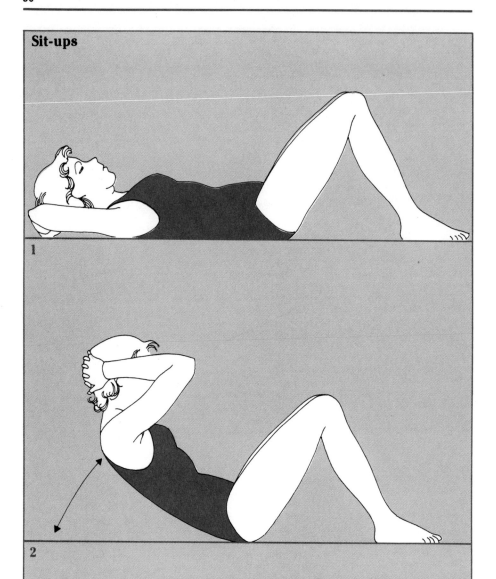

1. Start on your back with your legs bent and your knees raised. Put your hands either behind your head or to your temples, with your elbows out to the side. Tuck your chin.

2. Keeping your feet flat on the floor and maintaining your pelvic tilt, curl up, starting with your shoulders, then your shoulder blades, then your midback, and finally your lower back. Then slowly return to your starting position. Repeat this at least six times.

Advanced leg raises *Good* Ⓧ

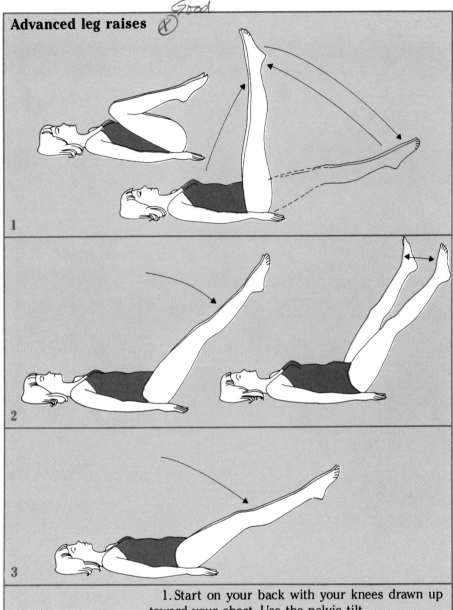

1

2

3

1. Start on your back with your knees drawn up toward your chest. Use the pelvic tilt.

Straighten your legs upward, then lower them toward the floor. At 1 foot from the floor, stop, and bring them back up. Repeat.

2. As a variation, lower your legs to a 45-degree angle. Hold them there and, keeping them straight, spread them apart, then bring them back together again. Raise your legs to the starting position. Repeat.

3. For added strengthening, try lowering your legs to a 30- or 20-degree angle.

Advanced sit-ups ✓

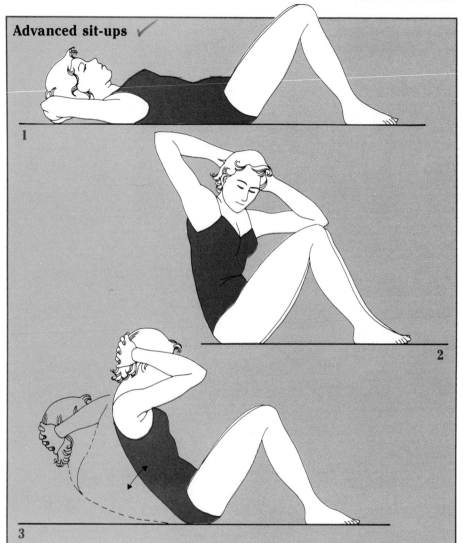

1. Start on your back with your legs bent and your knees raised. Put your hands behind your head and tuck your chin in.

2. One sit-up variation is to try to touch your left elbow to your right knee as you curl up and then repeat, touching your right elbow to your left knee. Repeat each combination six times.

3. The simplest and perhaps most difficult variation on the sit-up sounds easy—don't sit all the way up, and don't go all the way back down. Only curl up to about 70 degrees, hold this for a moment, then uncurl to about 20 degrees, keeping your shoulders from touching the floor. This is difficult because you don't get to rest at either end of the movement.

Thigh exercises

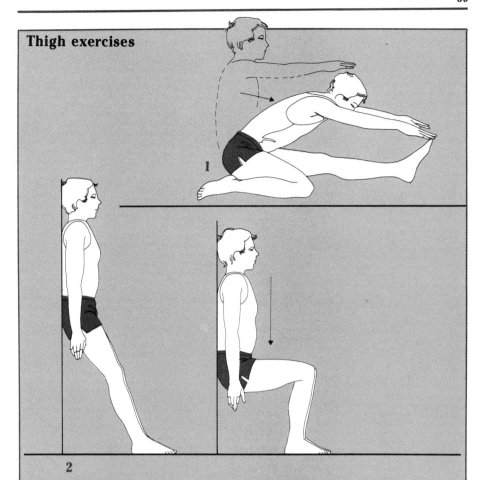

Stretched and strong thigh muscles will make maintaining the pelvic tilt easier.

1. To stretch your thigh muscles, use the "hurdler's stretch." Sit on the floor with one leg straight out in front of you and the other laid flat and bent at your side. Bend forward slowly and try to touch the toes on the leg straight out in front of you. Repeat this six times, alternating your legs.

2. To strengthen your thigh muscles, use a downhill skier's exercise. Stand with your back flat against a wall, with your feet 2½ feet out from the wall. Then slowly sit down, as if on an imaginary chair, until your thighs are parallel to the ground. Hold this for a slow count of six, then repeat. The average person has trouble maintaining the seated position for more than thirty seconds. Downhill skiers, who must maintain a similar position for the length of a race, can hold the position for 5 minutes.

Neck strengthening

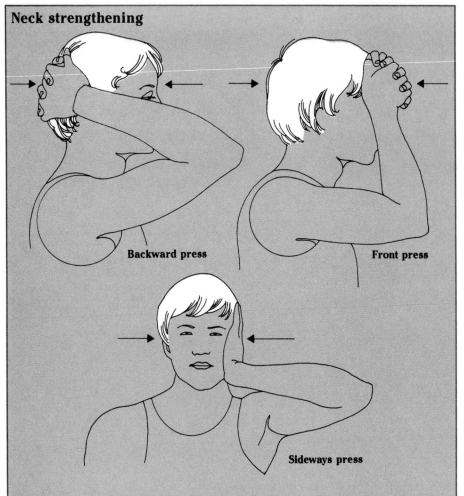

Backward press

Front press

Sideways press

These three basic exercises strengthen your neck muscles. They're all variations on one principle—isometrics, in which you push against yourself. In all of these exercises, you start by sitting upright, with proper posture, in a chair. In the *backward press*, you clasp your fingers behind your head and press them toward your head as you press your head backward. Hold for a slow count of six. In the *front press*, you put the palms of your hands against your forehead and press them toward your head as you press your head forward. In the *sideways presses*, you put your left hand above your left ear and press it toward your head as you press your head against it for a count of six; then repeat, using your right hand above your right ear. Don't overdo any of these—if your neck or head quivers, you're overdoing it.

Neck and shoulder relaxation

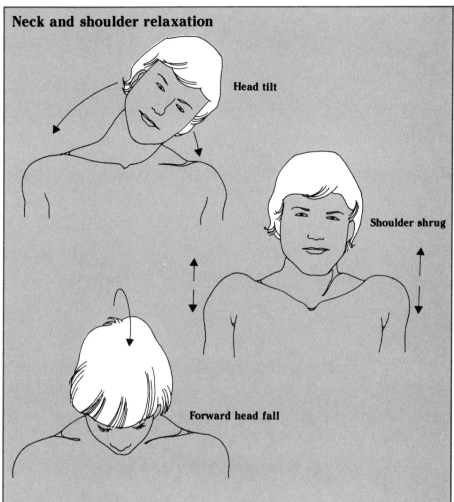

Head tilt

Shoulder shrug

Forward head fall

Done from a sitting position, these simple exercises work out your neck and shoulder kinks. First, tilt your head from side to side, as if you were trying to touch your ears to your shoulders. Next, let your head fall forward, then look from side to side. When working out your neck, *do not* let your head fall back. That only overarches your cervical spine, which isn't good for it.

To relax your shoulders, try an exaggerated shrug, bringing your shoulders as far up toward your ears as you can, holding them there for a few moments, then relaxing them. Also thrust your shoulders back as far as you can, as if you were trying to touch your shoulder blades together. Hold that for a moment, then relax. Then thrust them forward as far as you can, hold for a moment, then relax.

Hip extension

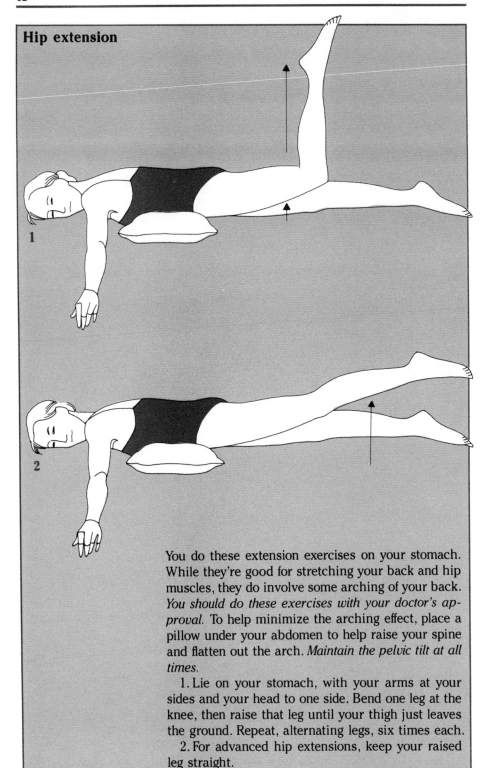

You do these extension exercises on your stomach. While they're good for stretching your back and hip muscles, they do involve some arching of your back. *You should do these exercises with your doctor's approval.* To help minimize the arching effect, place a pillow under your abdomen to help raise your spine and flatten out the arch. *Maintain the pelvic tilt at all times.*

1. Lie on your stomach, with your arms at your sides and your head to one side. Bend one leg at the knee, then raise that leg until your thigh just leaves the ground. Repeat, alternating legs, six times each.

2. For advanced hip extensions, keep your raised leg straight.

Arm and trunk extension

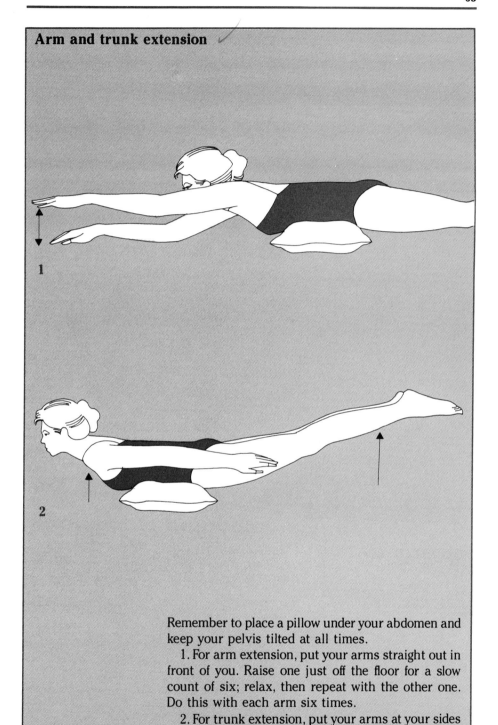

Remember to place a pillow under your abdomen and keep your pelvis tilted at all times.

1. For arm extension, put your arms straight out in front of you. Raise one just off the floor for a slow count of six; relax, then repeat with the other one. Do this with each arm six times.

2. For trunk extension, put your arms at your sides and slowly raise your head and shoulders until they just leave the floor. Hold this for a count of six, then repeat six times.

Perform all these exercises slowly, smoothly, and conscientiously. A simple regimen combining a variety of these exercises should take no more than 10 minutes a day. Even doing them twice a day—a good idea when you're starting out—won't take a great deal of time.

These exercises should not be an arduous workout, but a gradual strengthening and limbering up. Incorporate these exercises into the warm-up and cool-down exercises you perform for whatever sport or activity you engage in. Many people come to look forward to these exercises as a way to relax and relieve tension.

They are most important a few weeks after back pain, for the spasms will have weakened your muscles, which you must strengthen again.

Do these exercises once a day, every day. After a few months of doing so, you just might find that your back isn't bothering you as much as it used to.

Back Care

Atten-shun!

One trouble with trying to achieve proper posture is that popular ideas of how to stand are confused. Many people associate proper posture with the ramrod-straight back and thrust-back shoulders of soldiers on parade. This stance may do well for troops on review but doesn't do any good for the back. A soldier's rigid stance can become uncomfortable very quickly; proper posture should make you feel relaxed.

Y ou can prevent most back problems by learning how to stand, sit, work, and relax in ways that will help your back.

Proper posture

The goal of proper posture is to distribute your body weight evenly and avoid muscle strain. This means standing with your head up, your shoulders straight, and your pelvis tilted.

• Stand with your head up, your eyes looking straight ahead, and your chin in (jutting out your chin puts an uneven load on your neck). Your aim is to balance your head directly over your spine so that the weight is transmitted straight down the spine's length.

• Keep your shoulders straight. Don't let them slump forward. You may feel more relaxed that way, but doing so puts strain on a group of muscles across your back and shoulders (a common cause of muscle tension headaches). Pushing your shoulders all the way back in a military posture isn't the answer—that strains other muscles and throws your head forward over your neck, out of balance. The correct position lies in between, with your shoulders neither bowed forward nor pulled back too far.

• Tilt your pelvis. The foundation of proper posture is the pelvic tilt (see page 46). By tightening your

Look ahead

A common postural error is walking, sitting, or standing with the head bowed to any degree—your head needn't be at an eyes-to-the-ground angle to put unnecessary stress on your neck. As much as possible, keep your eyes looking straight ahead. Looking ahead tilts your head back to the correct position, directly over your spine.

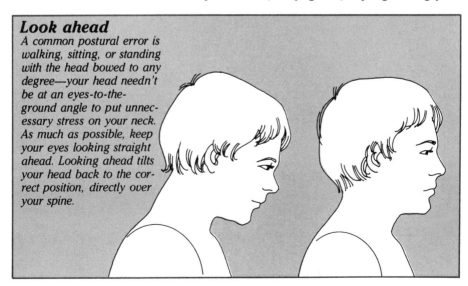

Helping your back

By nature, we do many things for our back. Bar patrons have long known they can stand longer with one foot raised—the reason many bars have a railing running 6 inches off the floor the length of the bar. When you cross your legs while sitting, you raise one leg higher than your hips, easing your back. When you put your feet up to relax, you're again raising your knees above your hips. And the most common sleeping position—the fetal position, which comes to us so naturally—is also just about the best position for your back.

High heels and back trouble

Wearing high heels can not only give you sore feet but also may contribute to a lower backache. High heels put your feet on a downward slant. Your weight is pulled forward by gravity, but you don't lean forward because your back automatically compensates for this forward pitch. You lean backward—increasing the natural curve of your lower back (the lumbar lordosis). Increasing this curve can strain your back muscles.

To prevent back problems and especially if you already have back problems, wear low heels whenever possible. If you must wear high heels, wear them when you know you won't be standing for long.

stomach muscles and pulling in your buttocks, you tilt your pelvis toward your back, which gives support to your lower spine. This distributes your weight more evenly in your lumbar region—your lower back—and balances the work of the muscles that support and move your spine.

If you must stand for long periods—if you work in a store, for example—you can tilt your pelvis back and take strain off your lower back by placing one foot on a stool, chair, or other object (select something about 6 inches high).

If you can't find something to rest a foot on, shift your weight back and forth from leg to leg; when standing straight, balance your body weight evenly on both feet.

If you sense tightness or soreness in your back, slowly crouch into a position like that used by baseball catchers. Done for a few moments, this can stretch the muscles in your lower back and stop the joints from stiffening.

If you must bend over to work on something, don't bend at the waist; instead, bend your knees.

Walking

Maintain proper posture while walking and keep your weight directly over your spine and pelvis. Resist the tendency to lean forward. Avoid high heels: they throw your body off balance and put uneven stresses on your spine. Low-heeled walking shoes are best.

Sitting

Sitting puts a much greater load on your back than standing or walking. If you lean forward—as you might when working over a desk—you increase the stress on your back. Try to sit in such a way that your hips are 6 inches or so in front of your shoulders. This makes the chair absorb some of the weight of your upper body, taking it off your lower back.

The chair you select is important, particularly if your job requires you to sit for many hours each day. Avoid soft, cushioned chairs, and select a firm chair that has enough room in the seat to permit you to shift your weight and has a back that curves in to support your lower back. Armrests allow you to distribute your weight more easily; using the armrests when you stand will also save your back some stress. The best office chair is one that tilts, swivels, and has an adjustable height. Adjust the height of the chair

Back aids

The issue of proper posture has been confused by a deluge of devices—from heelless shoes to backless chairs—designed to aid our backs. Doctors will tell you that posture—how you sit, stand, sleep, walk—is far more important than any equipment. People often spend years searching for the "right" chair or bed. While some beds and chairs are better for you than others, sitting with correct posture on a poor chair is better than sitting incorrectly on a great one.

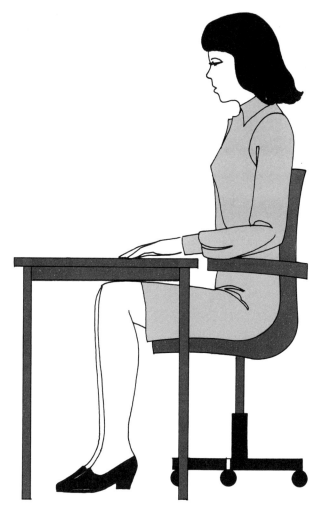

so that when you place your feet flat on the floor your knees are slightly higher than your hips; you should be able to slide your hand between your thigh and the seat. If you can't adjust the height of the chair, use something—a box or small stool—as a footrest. Raising your knees higher gives relief to your lower back. Crossing your legs occasionally will also tilt your pelvis back, relieving strain on the small of your back.

If the chair back doesn't offer any support for your lower back, try placing a small pillow between the chair and your lower back. This will relieve some strain.

Check your desk, too. If it's too low, you'll bend forward as you work; if it's too high, you'll lean back.

To avoid bending forward, sit as close as you can to your desk (your chair's armrests should be low enough to slide under the top of the desk).

When sitting on the ground, you can help your back by crossing your legs or bringing your knees up toward your chest and leaning back against something—a wall, a tree, or even the back of a friend.

Driving

When driving, make sure your seat is fairly low (not so low you have to strain to see the road, of course) and up close to the wheel; your knees should be at about your hip level and you should be able to reach the pedals without fully extending your leg. This lets you keep your arms and legs bent as you drive, a much more relaxed position. Driving with your legs straight can hurt your lower back; driving with your arms straight out in front of you tires your shoulders and your neck. Stay close to keep your arms, shoulders, and neck relaxed—this is the position to assume when performing any work. You may find that a small cushion placed behind your lower back will help relieve strain there. Stop occasionally during long drives, get out, and walk around.

If you're tired, don't slump in a chair: lie down.

Sleeping

Lying down is the least stressful position for your back. When you're sleeping, your back is spared the weight of your body; the pressure on your vertebrae is released, and your back's muscles can relax. Even so, some positions for sleeping are better than others.

Sleeping on your stomach isn't good for your back. No matter how hard your mattress, this position bends your body, sinking your stomach into the mattress and overarching your back. You also have to twist your head to sleep on your stomach, and that can lead to a stiff neck. If you must sleep on your stomach, put a pillow under your abdomen to raise and somewhat flatten your back's arch.

The two best sleeping positions are on your back and on your side. While sleeping on your back, rest your head on some kind of neck support—a pillow— and have your legs bent and your knees raised. To keep your knees raised while you sleep, put a couple

Don't arrive with a backache
On long trips by plane, train, or bus, place a small pillow or rolled-up towel behind your lower back to add support. If the seat doesn't have a footrest, put your feet up on a briefcase or small bag. Get up and walk around and stretch at least every 30 minutes. If your back gets sore—and you can find the room—try stretching out by adopting the baseball catcher's crouch: curl over to stretch your back even further.

of pillows under them, perhaps wrapped in a sheet so they won't move as you sleep. While wonderful for your back, this position can be hard to maintain through the night.

The best position is on your side with your legs curled up—the fetal position. Rest your head on a pillow to keep your spine straight; don't use too many pillows, for this will only bend your neck. You may also put a pillow between your knees, to keep from restricting the lower leg's circulation and to keep from twisting your spine with the drop of your upper leg. You can also support your upper arm on a pillow or two to keep from straining your neck and shoulder muscles.

Two good sleeping positions

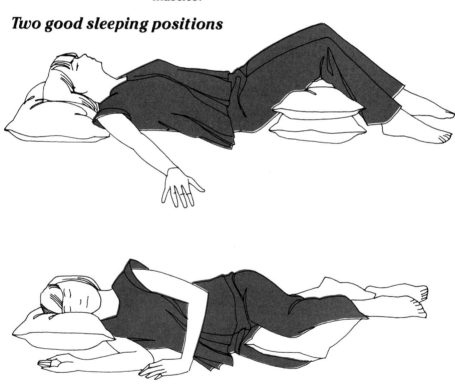

Ranking the positions

Here are the eight most common positions, ranked from best to worst according to how much pressure they put on your lower back:

1. Sleeping on your back
2. Sleeping on your side
3. Standing upright
4. Sitting upright
5. Standing, slouched forward slightly
6. Sitting, slouched forward slightly
7. Standing, bending forward
8. Sitting, leaning all the way forward

Your mattress

Some doctors argue that concern for mattress hardness is more the result of successful marketing by mattress companies than an indication that soft mattresses give you lower back pain. A mattress should give support, but as long as you sleep with your knees bent, the mattress can be as soft as you like. If you'd like to try a firmer bed, just place a sheet of plywood under your mattress.

Pillows, too, have been the subject of much debate. Some doctors claim you shouldn't sleep with any pillows, and some argue that pillows supply needed support. The specially designed neck-support pillows now available support the arch in your neck, an arch usually flattened when you sleep on normal pillows. When you sleep on your side, such pillows keep your head up and your neck free from strain. However, a rolled-up towel under your neck can do the job one of these pillows does when you're on your back, and almost any pillow will suffice when you're sleeping on your side.

How backpackers pack

Backpackers have long known a good trick for carrying heavy loads—they transfer some of the weight off their backs. Backpacks often have a waist belt that can be tightened around the hips. That way the pack rests not only on the shoulder straps but on the waist belt. Some of the pack's weight is thus taken off the back and placed directly on the hips and legs.

Lifting and carrying

Factory workers have long known that they have to take care of their backs. Lifting a heavy or even not-so-heavy object the wrong way can cause trouble. One bad lift can cause a muscle spasm in your back; several bad lifts can lead to chronic back problems.

For many decades, the walls of factories and warehouses across the country have been adorned with posters showing the proper way to lift things. We should all have one of those posters, because the mover who lugs refrigerators all day isn't the only person who needs to be concerned with his back. Anyone who carries groceries or moves a typewriter from one desk to another or picks up and carries any object should know the proper way to lift and carry things.

The basic principle behind lifting is "easy does it." Make the job as easy as possible, and make sure you can handle the job before you begin lifting. With heavy objects, try to find a way to move them rather than lift and carry them. You might put a heavy chair or sofa on a dolly. Or you can slip a carpet or heavy blanket under a heavy or large object and pull it across

Stay close to your work

Working with your arms over your head can tire your back and strain arm, shoulder, and neck muscles. If you must work on something above your head, try to raise yourself to the work's level. For example, if you're painting a ceiling, use a long-handled roller and paint a portion of the ceiling out in front of you, not directly over your head, so that you don't have to look straight up and bend your neck and back. When Michelangelo painted the ceiling of the Sistine Chapel, he didn't stand on the scaffolding—he lay down on his back on the scaffolding, giving his back a rest (and the world an art masterpiece).

the floor (this also prevents floor scratching). You can "walk" refrigerators and other large appliances across a floor—rock them back and forth on their corners, moving them forward with each rock and turn.

If an object is an awkward shape, try to make it less so. A flat rectangle, such as a box containing an overcoat, may be too large to carry comfortably under your arm, but if you use a loop of rope or heavy string to fashion a makeshift handle, the chore becomes manageable. Indeed, a length of rope can be tied around the most awkward object to make it easier to grab.

The object's location can also pose problems. The worst motion for your back is a twisting, shearing motion. This occurs when you bend over and twist or turn while lifting something. Some of the classic examples of this motion are difficult to avoid: how else can a parent lift a baby out of a crib, and how else can a golfer get golf clubs out of a car trunk? You can't perform such lifts properly—that is, you can't keep your back straight and lift with your legs.

(text continued on page 74)

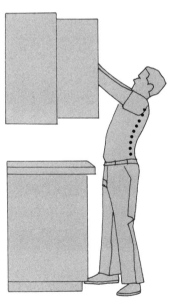

**Reaching that strains
your back**

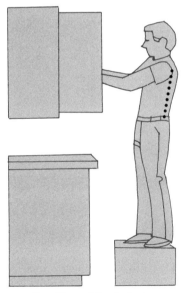

Reaching without strain

Letting leverage help you

The reason you should hold objects close to your body when lifting or carrying them is based on a principle of physics: leverage. If you hold an object out at arm's length, your arms are being used in a levering action, with your body as the pivot point. This makes the object seem much heavier than if it were held close to your body. You can demonstrate this for yourself by holding a thick book straight out. You'll have trouble holding it out there for very long. As you bring it in toward your body, you'll notice that it seems to get lighter.

Follow these steps when lifting or carrying objects:

1. Size up the job. Can you manage it? Can you grasp the object firmly? Test the weight of the load before you lift it; get help if you have any doubts. Are other items in the way?

2. Keep your back straight. This means both flattening out your lower back with a pelvic tilt and keeping your back vertical, making sure you don't bend over as you lift.

3. Stand near the object to be lifted and bend at the knees, not at the waist. When picking up anything—even a piece of paper—that's lower than your

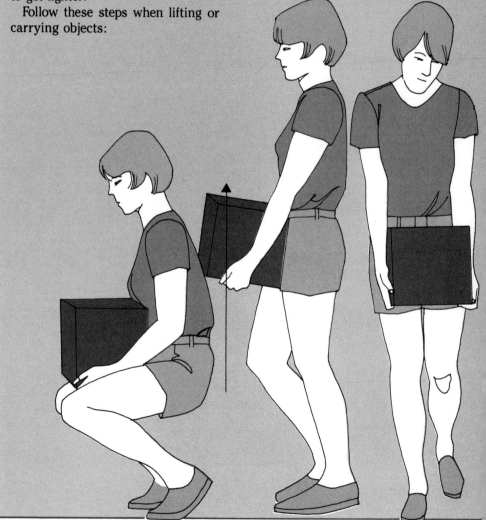

waist, don't bend over to get it; bend your knees and squat down close to the object you want to lift.

4. Grasp the object firmly. Make sure you've got a good grip before lifting. A sudden slip can throw you off balance and open your back to a muscle pull or worse.

5. Lift with your legs, not with your back. Your leg muscles are stronger than your back muscles. Stand up slowly.

6. Don't twist your back. If you want to turn as you hold the object, use your feet and turn your entire body.

7. Hold the object close while lifting and carrying it. This puts less pressure on your lower spine than does holding it away from you.

8. Don't lift heavy objects located above your shoulders. If you try to pick up something high in a cupboard or on top of a bookshelf, your back will arch, and your weight load will be unbalanced. When you must get something up high, use a chair or stepladder to bring yourself up to its level.

9. Follow the same rules when setting down objects. Remember to bend your legs, not your back.

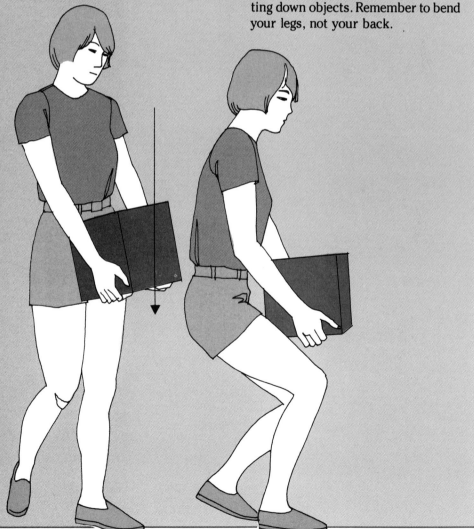

Therefore, you must think ahead and not get yourself into the situation: the parent should get a crib with sides that can be lowered or folded down; the golfer should put the clubs in the car's back seat so they can simply be pulled out instead of lifted.

Use your legs when you lift

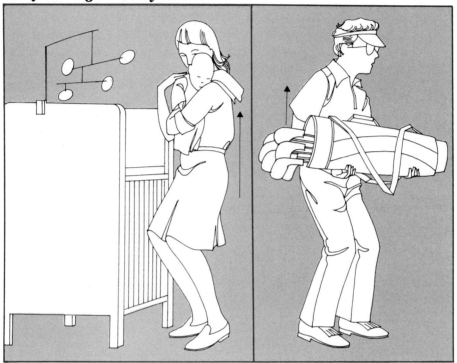

Don't make the mistake of following these rules for big objects but ignoring them for small, light objects. The basic rules apply to lifting and carrying even the smallest, lightest object. Bending over even to tie your shoes isn't a good idea. You may be tempted to ignore the rules when you pick up your briefcase or a basket of laundry, but even these objects can be a big load for your back when you're bent over. You'll avoid all problems by remembering to bend at the knees, keep your back straight, and lift with your legs.

A good way to make sure you do all your lifting and carrying the proper way is to maintain the pelvic tilt. Not only will the tilt flatten the arch in your back, evenly distribute your weight, and give added strength and support to your spine, but it will also help you remember your basic lift rule. Why? You can't bend your back much or twist as you lift when you keep those muscles tight.

Special concerns of pregnant women

If you're pregnant, you're probably very much aware of your back. The baby's weight can further exaggerate your lumbar curve, causing you a great deal of discomfort. To limit this, avoid gaining more weight than your doctor says is acceptable. You should also practice the pelvic tilt as often as necessary to ease the pressure on your lower back. You'll probably be able to perform most of the back exercises in this book (see pages 45 to 64); consult with your doctor first, of course.

If you can, sleep on your back with your knees bent. But if your back hurts, relieve the ache by performing the flexion maneuver (see page 35).

Throughout pregnancy and especially while breast-feeding, keep your calcium intake adequate. A lot of calcium goes into making milk, and if your body doesn't find the calcium in the food you eat, it will start to draw it from reserves in your organs and tissues and then your bones. Calcium depletion in the bones makes them porous and brittle (see pages 14 and 15 for a further discussion of this disease, osteoporosis).

Special concerns of the elderly

The primary targets of osteoporosis are people over age 60, with women running a higher risk than men. But osteoporosis begins its course at an early age, so we must all keep our calcium intake levels up from our early twenties on. Osteoporosis-weakened vertebrae are prone to fracture.

If you're elderly, be sensible in your activities, but be sure to keep active and stick with your exercises. While arthritic changes in your spine may limit your flexibility, you should still perform the exercises to keep your joints loose and your muscles stretched and strong. Exercise is also important because it promotes calcium replacement in the bones.

Big stomachs
Take a look at an Olympic weight lifter; you'll probably notice a very large stomach. Why would an Olympic athlete have such a huge stomach? Don't be fooled. Not all of that stomach is fat. Much of it is muscle—overdeveloped abdominal muscles—needed by the lifter to flatten the arches in his back and keep his spine rigid while lifting the extreme weights.

8 Alternative Therapies

Have you noticed that the more you find out about a subject, the more you find that you still have to learn? This is certainly true with research into back problems. As experts have learned more and more about the back, they've had to discard many theories and assumptions about back problems that seem perfectly logical.

Experts still argue about whether back pain is caused by irritated facet joints, a disk's core bulging into its outer walls, or a pinched nerve. We still don't know exactly what goes wrong in the back; nor do we know exactly what should be done to remedy back problems. A treatment that, by medical logic, should succeed very often won't. What we do know is that some treatments work better than others.

Conventional medicine provides two routes—depending on the diagnosis—for the severe back pain sufferer. Most patients with back problems—those with irritated facet joints and herniated disks that haven't completely ruptured—take one route: bed rest to see them through the acute phase followed by exercise, maintenance of proper posture, and general back care. The second route—surgery—is applicable only to those with a ruptured disk, with a free-floating fragment pressing against a nerve root.

This lack of options is frustrating for many people. We have high expectations of medicine—we expect doctors to be able to cure any and all diseases. But even though we know a great deal about the back and the possible causes of back problems, our expectations can't always be met. These unmet expectations lead many people to alternative therapies. Some alternative therapies relieve back pain, but most are still controversial. Here are some of the best-known alternative therapies.

Chymopapain injection

Chymopapain injection is the newest and most controversial of the nonsurgical treatments for disk problems. Chymopapain, an enzyme extracted from the

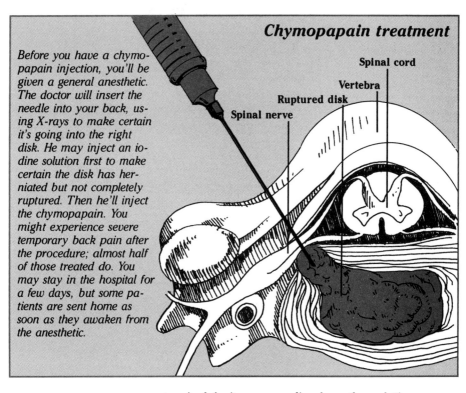

Chymopapain treatment

Before you have a chymopapain injection, you'll be given a general anesthetic. The doctor will insert the needle into your back, using X-rays to make certain it's going into the right disk. He may inject an iodine solution first to make certain the disk has herniated but not completely ruptured. Then he'll inject the chymopapain. You might experience severe temporary back pain after the procedure; almost half of those treated do. You may stay in the hospital for a few days, but some patients are sent home as soon as they awaken from the anesthetic.

Spinal cord

Vertebra

Ruptured disk

Spinal nerve

tropical fruit papaya, dissolves the gelatinous contents of a disk—the disk's core or nucleus. Chymopapain is therefore used for a herniated disk that presses against a nerve. When the nucleus is removed, the pressure against the disk or nerve is relieved.

Chymopapain injection is touted as a faster, less expensive alternative to surgery. Some back experts claim it could eliminate much back surgery; others say it's worthless.

Actually, this treatment isn't new. It was introduced in the United States 20 years ago by Dr. Lyman Smith of Elgin, Ill. After learning of the substance's properties, he devised an injectable form of the enzyme and used it to treat patients with herniated disks. By 1974, nearly 10,000 Americans had received injections of chymopapain. In 1974, however, the Food and Drug Administration (FDA) banned the use of the enzyme when research failed to confirm its beneficial effects. But chymopapain wasn't banned in Canada or Europe, and many American back sufferers made pilgrimages to get injections of the drug. Later FDA research showed chymopapain to be effective, and in 1982 its use in the United States was again allowed.

Controversy still surrounds chymopapain. Those who support it claim that it's less expensive, more successful, and simpler than surgery. They claim that chymopapain therapy is successful for 75% of the patients who undergo it, whereas surgery is successful for only 60% of patients.

Opponents of chymopapain injection argue that although it may be less expensive than surgery, it isn't simpler and doesn't have a higher rate of success. They point out that, like surgery, chymopapain injection is performed in a hospital with the patient under anesthesia and that the patient requires hospital convalescence. As for the success rate, some surgeons dispute the 75% success rate of chymopapain but do admit that three quarters of the people who receive the injections into herniated disks feel less pain afterward. Furthermore, many surgeons dispute the low 60% success rate assigned to surgery. They argue that when surgery is limited to the removal of a free-floating fragment from a ruptured disk—the only case where surgery is appropriate—the success rate is over 90%, far surpassing the success rate of chymopapain treatment.

Opponents also point to the dangers of chymopapain injection. One in 100 patients receiving chymopapain treatment suffers a severe allergic reaction, and of the 60,000 or so who have received it, 10 have died.

Is chymopapain treatment for you?
Chymopapain treatment isn't for everyone. If you have asthma or suffer from severe allergic reactions, you won't be permitted to undergo chymopapain treatment. People who've had spinal surgery in the past are also usually ruled out.

Even chymopapain's supporters acknowledge that it shouldn't be used in some instances, as when a disk has completely ruptured and a piece of its core has broken through the outer walls. But that's the instance that many surgeons say is the only one appropriate for surgery. Therefore, chymopapain injection really isn't an alternative to surgery: it can't be used in the one instance in which surgery can help.

Chiropractic

Chiropractic is a system of healing based on the theory that disease results from a lack of normal nerve function. According to chiropractic theory, a spine out of perfect alignment can cause problems throughout the body. The founder of chiropractic, Daniel Palmer, claimed that one day in Iowa in 1895 he cured a man's deafness by manipulating his spine. Such grand claims are rarely made of chiropractic these days. However, chiropractors do claim wonders from

That slipped disk,
again
A disk can't slip because it's firmly attached to the vertebrae above and below it. What does slipped disk mean then? It's a herniated disk, where the disk's core squeezes out (herniates), usually from a weakened part of the disk's outer shell. When this core material contacts a spinal nerve, pain results.

manipulating spinal joints to put disks and vertebrae back into their correct positions.

Regardless of chiropractors' claims, disks and vertebrae can't come out of position. Disks don't slip, and vertebrae rarely come out of alignment—and even if they did, you couldn't manipulate them from the surface with only the pressure of hands. Even surgeons who open up a back and lay their hands directly on a spine can't budge the vertebrae. Nevertheless, someone who has spinal manipulation by a chiropractor is likely to hear a loud crack. The sound isn't caused by a disk or vertebra popping back into place, however. The sound is similar to the one you make when you crack a knuckle—you pop a gas pocket that builds up in the joint.

Although chiropractors can't do all they claim, they still do some good. The manipulation can relax muscles and loosen stiff joints. Many people feel great relief after visiting a chiropractor. Such relief is usually only temporary—chiropractors can't do anything about the pain's cause.

One real concern about chiropractic is its extensive use of X-rays, exposing the patient to radiation. If you go to a chiropractor, say no to a full back X-ray. Also, while chiropractic is unlikely to harm you, if you see a chiropractor, also see a doctor; otherwise, you might let a treatable condition go untreated.

Traction

Traction uses a system of weights and pulleys to stretch your spine, relieving nerve root compression. While traction might provide you temporary relief, it accomplishes nothing permanent. As one surgeon has noted, traction is a good idea for people in the acute phase because it keeps them immobile and on their back.

Gravity inversion

A variation on traction, gravity inversion involves hanging upside down from your ankles, using either an elaborate contraption or special boots that can hook onto an overhead bar. The idea is that by relieving your vertebrae, disks, and joints of gravity's pressure, you're relieved of pain.

Initial claims that gravity inversion could stretch your spine and restore the spaces between vertebrae lost to disk degeneration were unfounded. However, gravity inversion isn't harmful to your back and can provide some relief because it stretches muscles and loosens joints. You can accomplish the same benefits with exercise.

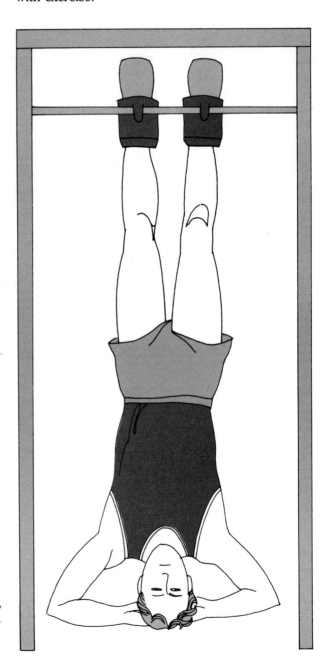

Gravity inversion
Some people use gravity-inversion equipment to perform exercises to strengthen leg and abdominal muscles (some doctors believe such upside-down exercises may be harmful to your back). You should never use gravity-inversion equipment alone—you may not be able to release yourself from your upside-down position.

Transcutaneous electrical nerve stimulation (TENS)

First was the theory of nerve blocks—that if you severed the nerve carrying the pain, the pain would cease. The relief, however, was only temporary, because, defying logic, the pain would return. Then came TENS. The theory here is that small zaps of electricity to the skin over the painful area—delivered from a small, strap-on device—can distract the brain from the pain, just as pressing a cut on a finger distracts and eases the hurt. Unfortunately, though TENS can cause initial relief, the body adjusts and the pain returns in a few weeks.

Do's and don'ts

The typical TENS user is the patient with chronic back pain. However, TENS is also effective after knee, hip, or back surgery; in phantom limb pain, rheumatoid arthritis, or neuralgias, TENS should not be used if the patient has a cardiac pacemaker. Safety during pregnancy hasn't been established.

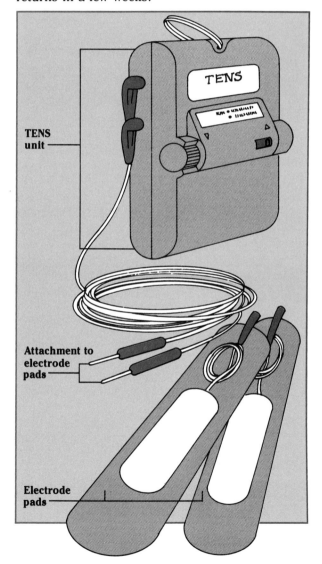

TENS unit

Attachment to electrode pads

Electrode pads

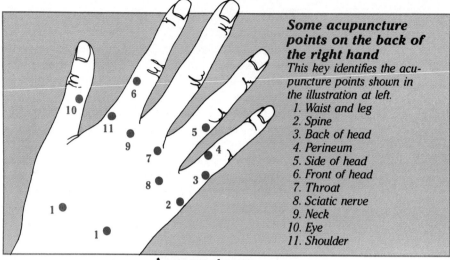

Some acupuncture points on the back of the right hand
This key identifies the acupuncture points shown in the illustration at left.
1. Waist and leg
2. Spine
3. Back of head
4. Perineum
5. Side of head
6. Front of head
7. Throat
8. Sciatic nerve
9. Neck
10. Eye
11. Shoulder

Acupuncture

Although at first greeted with skepticism, this ancient Chinese pain-relief method has gained credence in the West: it can work for many people. In this treatment, a technician inserts extremely thin needles into the patient's skin at various body points. (The needles have rounded ends so they push tissue apart rather than cut it.) Acupuncturists have charted over 1,000 of these body points, and by inserting typically 10 to 15 needles into a combination of points, they aim to relieve pain in a specific area.

The acupuncturist inserts the needles at various angles and to differing depths. The patient may feel a little discomfort at first. Then, as the acupuncturist turns, vibrates, or electrically stimulates the needles, the patient will experience other sensations, such as a dull throb, warmth, or light-headedness. Some patients get instantaneous relief from the treatment, some have to go back for several sessions before they find relief, and others will never respond to acupuncture.

How does acupuncture work? Some believe it works on the gate theory—that the needles' stimulation overpowers and overrides any pain messages going to the brain. Others believe that the needles may trigger the release of the body's own pain killers (endorphins).

A drawback to using acupuncture for back trouble is that it doesn't do anything to fix the underlying cause, whether it's disk degeneration or herniation. Also, the pain relief is only temporary. The patient will need regular treatments to keep the pain at bay.

Harmony

One important nondrug pain-relief technique that remains controversial is the ancient Chinese art of acupuncture. Some pain experts claim that acupuncture can relieve and prevent pain.

Acupuncture is based on the belief that disease results from an imbalance of the body's life force. To restore harmony, the practitioner inserts long, thin needles along body channels that affect the aching or diseased body part.

Because acupuncture involves skin penetration, it can damage or infect nerves or blood vessels. Therefore, licensing requirements in the United States remain stricter for acupuncture than for acupressure and chiropractic. In some states, the acupuncturist must be a licensed doctor.

Heat and cold therapy

From Roman baths to hot water bottles, we have been using heat therapy to relax us, soothe us, and ease our aches and pains. Why does heat provide pain relief? By increasing blood flow to damaged and inflamed tissues, heat may help carry off the by-products of the inflammation and so reduce the pain. By relaxing muscles, heat can ease tension. And, according to the gate theory, heat sensation may overpower and override the pain signals going to the brain.

Two types of heat therapy are superficial heat—the kind you get by pressing a hot water bottle to your back—and deep heat—applied by a trained practitioner with special equipment, usually ultrasound—which causes heat by vibrating deep muscle and bone.

The heat therapy most often used is superficial heat. It can be either dry heat—an electric heating pad or a heat lamp—or moist heat—a hot water bottle or a

Heat and cold therapy guidelines

Type	Temperature
HEAT	
Hot water bottle	Infants and geriatrics: 105 to 115 degrees F.; Adults: 115 to 125 degrees F.
Heating pad	Same as above
Infrared or ultraviolet lamp, depending on wattage	18 to 24 inches from skin
Gooseneck lamp	25 watts: 14 inches from skin; 40 watts: 18 inches; 60 watts: 24 to 30 inches
Hot compress	131 degrees F.
Hot soak	105 to 110 degrees F.
COLD	
Ice bag	50 to 80 degrees F., alternating 10 minutes on with 20 minutes off
Cold compress or pack	59 degrees F., alternating 10 minutes on with 20 minutes off
Chemical cold pack	50 to 80 degrees F., alternating 10 minutes on with 20 minutes off

Watch that heat!

Be careful with heat. You mustn't use too much heat (see the guidelines on page 83) or use any heat too long because burning is a risk (so be very careful if you're using a heating pad on skin where sensation is impaired). In fact, some doctors suggest that the best way to get the heat, if you can, is from the sun, using sunscreens to protect your skin.

Rolfing

Practitioners of rolfing attempt to relieve back pain and muscle tension by re-aligning body weight. They use rigorous, often painful physical manipulation and deep-tissue massage. The goal is to reduce back pain by helping the patient move more naturally with gravity.

Most people who perform rolfing schedule about 10 weekly 1-hour sessions. The considerable force and pressure used during a rolfing session can be painful. However, pain relief should follow the session.

hot, damp towel. Again, as with most of these pain-relief therapies, the relief is temporary, and, for the most part, the therapy does nothing to affect the pain's cause. Heat therapy can, however, affect one cause of pain: tense and spastic muscles.

Cold therapy is not effective for the temporary relief of long-term aches and pains. It does work, however, right after an injury because it can reduce swelling and inflammation. Cold seems to work two ways: by reducing the number of pain signals that go to the brain and by overpowering the sensation of pain.

You can apply cold in a number of ways. You can put ice cubes in a plastic bag, wrap the bag in a towel, and then press it against the injured areas. Or you can soak a towel in ice water, then wring it out and apply it to the sore area. You should never apply the cold for more than 10 minutes at a time or you'll risk frostbite and ice burns.

Cold therapy is appropriate only for those who have suffered muscle injury, since the cold can be used to reduce swelling, inflammation, and pain. The cold will not penetrate deep enough to affect the cause of the back pain, and it won't reduce facet joint inflammation or disk swelling.

Massage

Massage can bring a great deal of relief and relaxation. It may relieve pain by overpowering the pain signals going to your brain (the gate theory). Human touch is also comforting.

Because of the many muscles serving them, the back and the neck are good massage sites. To give a massage, have the person lie on his stomach, with a pillow or rolled up towel under his abdomen to support his lower back, and have him raise his arms and lie with his head to one side. Make sure your hands are warm before you begin. Use oil or lubricant, which you should also warm, so that your hands move smoothly over the skin.

Start at the spine's base and move up, concentrating on the sore or hurt area. Select from these four basic techniques:

- Use your thumbs.
- Place one hand over the other to give extra pressure.
- Knead with your thumbs and fingers.
- Chop with the sides of your hands.

Make your strokes firm, deliberate, even, and smooth. Make the transfer from one stroke to another smooth and continuous, and keep your hands on the person's back at all times. If the patient indicates pain, stop. Finish the massage with long strokes, from the base of the spine to the skull, gradually easing your pressure.

While massage can't treat the cause of common backache or provide anything more than temporary relief from back pain, it can greatly relax and ease a back sufferer's tension. For those having trouble getting to sleep because of their back pain, a massage can be an effective sedative.

Four basic massage motions

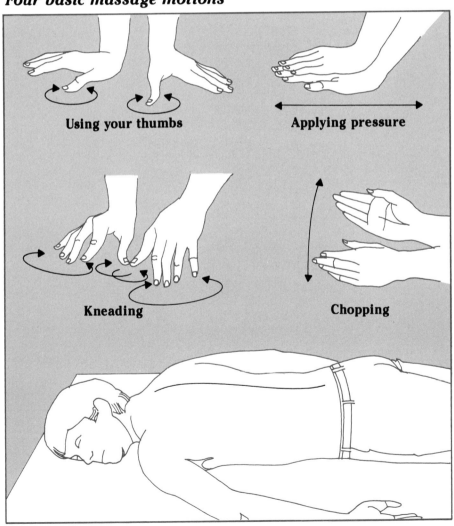

Using your thumbs

Applying pressure

Kneading

Chopping

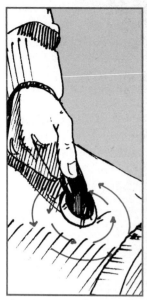

A technician will move the metal applicator in a circular motion over the muscles needing relaxation.

Ultrasound

Ultrasound can massage and heat tissue and muscle deep below the skin. It uses very low, subaudible sound waves that a technician directs into your body toward the affected area. The low sound waves vibrate and heat the tissue and muscle. This massage can relax the muscles and relieve pain. Like all the other pain relief methods cited here, ultrasound does nothing to affect the pain's cause and its pain relief is temporary. Also, ultrasound generally must be administered by trained practitioners, which means that a series of pain treatments can be expensive. Chiropractors frequently use ultrasound.

Hypnosis

Hypnosis has been practiced for over 200 years; yet we still know little about it and how it works. We know these four facts, though:
- Contrary to popular belief, hypnosis doesn't induce a sleeping state, but rather, a state of heightened concentration, where distractions are minimized and the mind is focused.
- People won't do anything under hypnosis that they wouldn't normally do.
- A patient is in no danger of "not waking up" because he's not asleep in the first place.
- You can probably learn self-hypnosis.

No one knows how hypnosis relieves pain. It doesn't trigger the release of endorphins, the body's own pain relievers. But it may activate the subconscious mind to hold back pain signals from the conscious mind.

However it works, hypnosis can be used in several ways for pain control and relief:
- to block the awareness of pain
- to substitute a different sensation—warmth or tingling, for example—for the pain
- to move the pain from the patient's back to a smaller area, such as a finger, where the pain is easier to cope with
- to distort time perception so that pain-free periods seem longer than painful ones
- through dissociation—the patient learns to separate himself from the pain.

The advantages of hypnosis-induced pain relief are that, if successful, the relief can be long-term, and, because hypnosis gives the patient a sense of pain control, it can lessen his anxiety, which may have worsened the pain in the first place. The drawbacks to the treatment? It's expensive, it doesn't work for everybody, and it can take a long time for the patient to become trained in the procedure. Two larger problems are that hypnosis may trigger anxiety reactions, and that successful pain suppression may hide an undiagnosed medical problem.

For back sufferers with chronic back pain, hypnosis can provide long-term, drug-free relief. As with all other methods of pain relief, however, it can do nothing to affect the pain's causes.

Biofeedback

For a long time, experts thought that such bodily functions as heart rate, blood pressure, and body temperature were automatic, involuntary, and beyond conscious control. However, just as a sense of panic can bring about changes in heart rate and blood pressure, so other thoughts and mental activities affect how our bodies behave—even how we experience pain.

In biofeedback, detectors hook up to various body parts to record temperature, skin reactions, blood pressure, heart rate, muscle tension, and brain waves. With the detectors in place, the patient tries to relax,

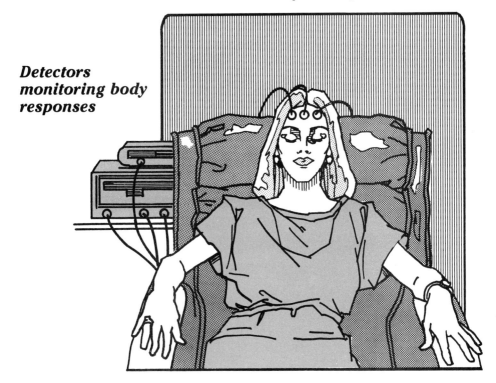

Detectors monitoring body responses

The placebo effect

A placebo is prescribed more for the patient's mental relief than for its actual effect. Although a placebo doesn't actually do anything to cure an ailment, the very act of taking a pill sometimes does the trick— the patient believes in the pill. Hypnosis, biofeedback, and other alternative methods may cure people in the same way.

using whatever technique he prefers. Most people select from autohypnosis, meditation, breathing exercises, suggestive imagery (such as conjuring up sunsets and waves), progressive muscle relaxation, or any combination of these. From the information gathered by the detectors, the person discovers what works to relax him.

After the person learns to relax by thinking of certain things, he can learn what mental patterns help control and ease pain. The drawbacks to this risk-free form of pain therapy are that it takes time to master and practice it, and it requires a high degree of patient motivation. Also, it may not work for everyone, and it won't affect the back pain's cause.

Your best choice

If an alternative therapy works for you, that's wonderful. The problems begin when someone scours the globe, going from one unsuccessful treatment to another in search of a cure. That's where overtreatment and potential problems come in.

During the past 50 years, we have devised better and better ways to care for and strengthen our backs. Even so, in basic ways we have to learn to live with our backs just as people did a half century ago. Your best choice is to lower your expectations from medicine and follow the advice in this book to avoid back problems. The truth is that the back is no simple thing, and back pain may never have a simple cure.

9

Common Questions about the Back

"Suddenly I have back problems. I've never had them before. What's happening?" You're just getting older. The degeneration of your disks begins when you're a teenager. Your spine changes and adapts to these changes throughout your life. Back pain comes when this process doesn't go as smoothly as it should. Back trouble is common. If you're a sufferer, you're one of 80 million in North America.

"What causes the pain?"

Mostly your muscles. With most back problems, the greatest pain comes from muscle spasms that attempt to immobilize your back, thus preventing further injury. Common backache is also predominantly muscular. But you can have other pain sources: the facet joints themselves cause pain. You may also have referred pain with some back problems. If the pain travels all the way down one leg, you probably have a pinched nerve.

"Why does it hurt so much?"

For a condition so common, back trouble seems to cause an inordinate amount of pain. However, your spine is so vital that your body wants to protect it, which includes sending messages of intense pain whenever anything goes wrong.

"Back trouble all stems from the day when man first started walking around upright, right?"

This commonly held belief seems to make sense. Before humans started walking around on two feet, some of the weight of our upper body was supported on the ground by our arms. But when we started to walk upright, all that weight had to be borne by the lower spine. As logical as this seems, however, walking around on two feet isn't at the root of back problems. Dogs, for example, are also prone to back pain, and many people get through life without one instance of back trouble.

"Will losing weight stop my back pain?"

Excess weight contributes to back pain. That doesn't mean losing weight is the entire answer, but you don't want to put any extra weight on your spine or increase your spine's curve, which stomach weight will do. Losing weight should be part of an entire program designed to give your back all the help you can.

"Do disks slip?"

Disks are so firmly attached to the vertebrae they're sandwiched between that they can't slip out of position. However, they can shrink, bulge, or even burst—all movements of a sort.

"My back hurt as I reached across the table. What did I do wrong?"

You didn't do anything wrong. The trouble started long before you reached. Your back in this situation is like a car tire with a bald spot. If you drive over a pothole, the tire may blow out. The weakness was there, waiting for the moment.

"The guy next to me—who's older, heavier, and has swayback—has no pain at all. How come?"

No one knows why certain people and not others are subject to back pain. Some people may have genetic weaknesses; others, who would seem to be more prone to trouble—such as the fellow you describe—go through life scott-free.

"How long do back problems last?"

The duration depends on the person and the severity of the problem. In general, pain from an irritated facet joint lasts from a few days up to 2 weeks. Pain from a nerve pinched by the fragment of a ruptured disk can last indefinitely—or until the fragment is removed.

"Do I need any special chairs, mattresses, or pillows?"

How you sit and sleep is more important than what you sit and sleep on. Even so, your chair should have certain characteristics (see pages 66 and 67), and you might sleep better on a firm mattress. Neck-support pillows are good. (A rolled-up towel can do the job just as well.)

"Can I still have sex?"

By all means. You may want to avoid anything that strains your back, but other than that, back pain needn't mean an end to sexual activity.

"What about sports?"

Do whatever you enjoy. If your sport hurts your back more than you're willing to put up with, think about switching sports. Swimming and cycling are two of the best sports for your back. Walking is great exercise, too. Whatever you do, do it often and don't worry about your back too much—you're not going to harm it.

"What rules can I follow?"

Follow these 10 rules to help avoid and to treat back problems:

1. Back trouble can't be cured, just controlled.
2. Get your back trouble properly diagnosed.
3. Get a second opinion.
4. The danger is overtreatment, not undertreatment.
5. Your pain is real, not in your head.
6. Stress, anxiety, and emotional upset can worsen back problems.
7. Most backache will pass with rest.
8. Exercise can help your back, but stop it if you hurt.
9. Proper posture and conscientious back care are vital.
10. Keeping your back healthy takes time, patience, and effort.

"Why is the back such a fragile, delicate body part?"

Actually, the back is remarkably strong and resilient, able to perform a variety of tasks. Considering the demands we make on our backs, they hold up surprisingly well.

"I had a bad fall as a child. That's what's behind my back pain now, right?"

Probably not. For a childhood injury to suddenly crop up again years later is highly unlikely. If your early fall did cause a chronic problem, you would have been troubled by it regularly ever since.

"Why does my neck hurt so much? Did I get a cold in my neck?"

Neck pain from a cold may seem to make sense, but, in truth, you can't get a cold there, nor is sleeping on your neck likely to cause the kind of pain and immobility that people feel when their neck muscles spasm. Probably you've got a little facet joint irritation that your neck wants to heal. A warm heating pad and a massage may help to relax the muscles, but don't try to stretch them or force your neck to move.

"How long should I wear my back brace?"

Wear it when you feel a need for added support and strength. But you should really look at it the same way you would a cane if you were recovering from a leg injury. After a time, you'd start to wean yourself from the cane, using it only for longer walks and eventually doing without it. You don't want to become dependent on a back brace since that can further weaken your muscles and make your back even more vulnerable. The best bet is exercise to strengthen your muscles, which are your own natural back brace.

"What's the difference between doctors, chiropractors, and osteopaths?"

Doctors receive degrees after 4 years of study at a recognized medical school. Osteopaths also study for 4 years, taking many of the same courses as doctors, with a concentration on bone study. Osteopaths may train as surgeons, in which case they perform spinal surgery. Chiropractors also study 4 years, concentrating on spinal anatomy. Their treatment is limited to what they accomplish by spinal manipulation.

"If my back doesn't get better, can't I always have surgery?"

Probably not. Only 1% of all back sufferers have a condition appropriate for surgical treatment—namely, a disk that has completely ruptured, causing a piece of its core to press against a nerve root. For almost all other cases, surgery isn't applicable.

"Everyone now says that back surgery is no good. Is this true?"

Back surgery can be very successful when it's used in appropriate situations—such as removing a ruptured disk fragment. Then, the success rate runs over 90%. Less prudent use of surgery lowers the overall back surgery success rate to roughly 60%.

"Do surgeons take out the whole disk when they operate? What goes in to replace it?"

First, a surgeon removes the disk fragment that presses against a nerve. Then he scrapes out the rest of the disk's core to ensure that the problem doesn't recur. You won't need anything added to replace the core because the disk quickly fills with scar tissue.

A final note

You should follow these two equally important but seemingly contradictory guidelines: think about your back at all times, but try not to think about it too much. In other words, give your back the attention it deserves—maintain good posture, lift things the right way, do your exercises, keep fit—but don't dwell on back problems. Dwelling on your back can often make matters worse—don't let your back dominate your life.

Index